# breathwork

# breathwork

## A 3-Week Breathing Program
to Gain Clarity, Calm, and Better Health

Valerie Moselle

Illustrations by Christian Papazoglakis

ALTHEA
PRESS

Interior and Cover Designer: Darren Samuel
Art Producer: Sara Feinstein
Editor: Nana Twumasi
Production Editor: Andrew Yackira
Illustrations: Christian Papazoglakis
Author photo courtesy of © Katherine Bree Walker Photography

ISBN: Print 978-1-64152-448-3
eBook 978-1-64152-449-0

*For my grandmother Annie,*
*who taught me to delight in everyday things.*

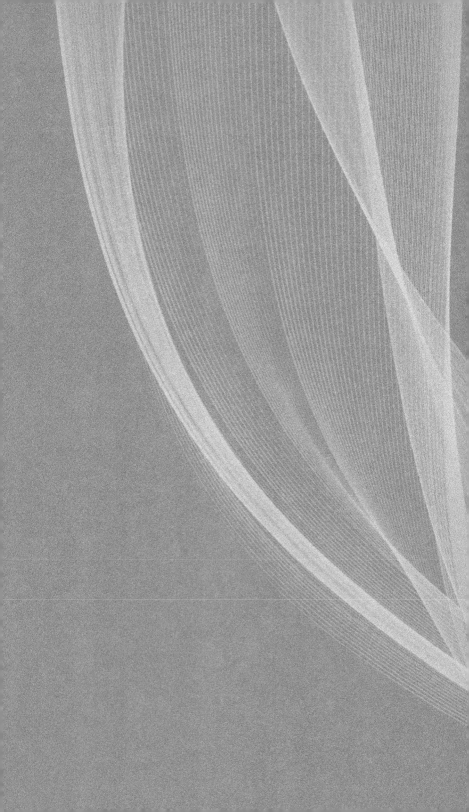

# Introduction

Our breath manifests within us as a physical embodiment of our life force, ever coming and going like waves. When we check to see if someone is alive, we listen for the breath. When our life force leaves us, it leaves with our last breath. Across cultures, breath is inspiration for art and poetry. It is relevant to us even beyond our physiological need for it.

Like many who have come to teach breathing, I began my relationship with formal techniques as a complement to postural yoga practice (*asana*). In the beginning, my teachers rarely spoke about the concrete benefits of conscious breathing. Lessons about breathing were given from a technical perspective, with the promise of long-term benefits based on metaphysical energy theory and elevated consciousness.

Yoga *pranayama* (breath control) is a way of redirecting *prana* (energy) in the body. Classically, the ultimate goal of yoga practice is to stir the energetic body in such a way that we become physically, psychologically, and energetically dislodged from our subjective experience of reality, along with all the assumptions that go with it. The promise is of a heightened state of awareness that enables us to see ourselves and the universe around us clearly. The objective is to find relief from the suffering that we each experience as part of our "mistaken" relationship with reality. Because of its association with yogic enlightenment, the reasons for practicing breath control remained in a nebulous realm of "someday" esoteric benefits that I couldn't yet comprehend.

But I did understand that we have a profound relationship with our breathing. We need our breath for moment-to-moment survival. If we stop breathing for even the shortest length of time, the desire for air becomes palpable and quickly overwhelms us. It is also clear that our breath changes to accommodate the immediate needs of our bodies. It becomes faster and fuller during physical exertion.

It naturally slows when we come into a place of stillness or intense mental focus. When we're waiting for something important to happen or witnessing an accident, we might hold our breath—suspended in a state of acute alertness. When startled, we gasp. When we're excited, our breath quickens. Both laughing and sobbing dramatically change our breathing.

Research shows that adapting our breathing can help us reduce stress, improve athletic performance, and strengthen our immune system. Breathing practices are commonly employed in the treatment of diseases such as diabetes, asthma, chronic obstructive pulmonary disease (COPD), and even cancer. Women giving birth are taught breathing techniques for pain management. Even Navy SEALs learn special breathing exercises to calm nerves and improve performance.

From my personal experience, as well as feedback from my students, I have come to see that developing our ability to gently, intuitively, and selectively shape our breathing enables us to more consciously engage with the complexity of life. The breath helps us stay clearer in the moment and be self-aware as we interact with our ever-changing world. But perhaps even more profound, diving deep into our breathing has the potential to reveal and heal hidden or repressed experiences, beliefs, or worldviews that inevitably limit our ability to authentically engage with everyone and everything around us.

Though the importance of the breath was first introduced to me through yoga study, my understanding of its value to everyday life—as a way of augmenting a moment in time, as a way of improving health, or as a way of processing emotion—became apparent only after years of what I have come to refer to as Breathwork. I often tell my students, "Yoga postures work on you from the outside in. The breath works on you from the inside out." In yoga, we can get caught up in the idea of the shapes we are making with our bodies rather than how we feel when we practice them. In contrast, breathing is acutely visceral. It happens in our chests, near our hearts, and also deep in our bellies; the sensations we associate with these regions are tender, personal, and poignant.

With this book I would like to encourage a playful approach to breath practice that emerges from a place of curiosity in you. I fully acknowledge that my experience of breathing might be entirely different from yours. A breath that fills me with joy might bring up anger for you. A technique that is challenging for me might feel as natural as yawning to you. So this book cannot be a "how to" with strict guidelines and rigid techniques for "correct" practice. Our breathing practices have the potential to awaken, heal, and inspire, but ultimately it is up to you to tune in to how best interact with them.

Over the next three weeks, I will support you in establishing a breathing practice that is both accessible and immediately rewarding. Your goal is simply to get to know your breath better and begin to recognize it as the tool that it is: a way to regularly access physical integration, cognitive awareness, and an enhanced connection with what is most meaningful to you.

Any daily practice needs to be something that we *want* to come back to again and again. If you've picked up this book in search of relief from something troubling you, such as anxiety or poor sleep, you are looking for immediate relief, not someday relief. While I can't promise a miracle or promise that breathing is the solution to anyone's problems, I can tell you that conscious breathing can be a natural mechanism for healing, available to every one of us at any time and in any place.

Many of the practices presented in this book are rooted in traditional techniques offered through various yoga and martial arts traditions. Most are practices that were introduced to me by my own teachers. I have omitted more complex or stimulating exercises that require the oversight of an experienced guide and have included only safe, accessible suggestions that can be explored by anyone of any age or physical ability.

The most challenging thing you're likely to face in the next three weeks will not be the practices themselves but simply showing up for them. Pausing during the day to integrate a new breathing practice can feel like one more "to-do." Life's unexpected challenges and surprises are likely to interfere. Consider approaching these weeks as you would approach a scientific experiment to see if daily breathing practices add value for you. The constant of the experiment is *consistent practice*. Your only other job is to observe whether Breathwork is making a difference.

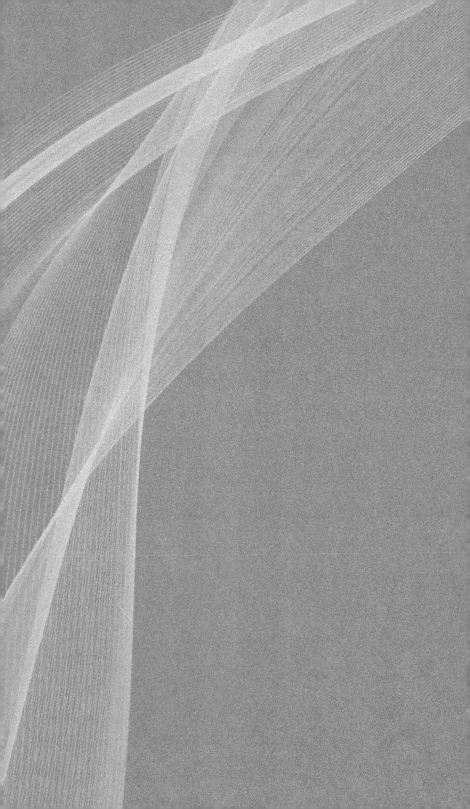

# PART ONE
## Before You Begin

## Chapter One

# It Begins with the Breath

Now we embark on our journey. In this chapter we'll learn about the physical mechanics of breathing and how developing breath awareness and properly employing certain techniques can help us live more satisfying and healthy lives. Most of us have simple needs; we want to sleep well, be reasonably comfortable in our bodies, feel clear and capable of accomplishing our tasks, and regularly experience a sense of meaning or purpose. Easy to say but not so easy to do, right? Let's take a look at the ways breathing can help us deal with a variety of issues, and then I'll give you an overview of the techniques we'll use.

# The Benefits of Breath

Perhaps you recall learning about breathing in your grade school biology class, in which case you remember that our lungs expose our blood to the air we breathe, and our blood picks up the oxygen molecules and moves them around our bodies. We never have to worry about forgetting to breathe (our bodies take care of it whether we pay attention or not), so the breath is often something we neglect. Yet proactive, conscious breathing has the potential to provide us with myriad benefits.

## Mood Management

How many times have you heard the suggestion to slow down and take a deep breath? It's a go-to for anyone in a crisis. We instinctively know that regulating disturbed breathing can help reduce anxiety, at least temporarily. Slowing and bringing awareness to our breathing also helps us tolerate other uncomfortable feelings, such as anger, over-excitement, and grief.

Between 2011 and 2014, an estimated one in nine Americans, including children, took antidepressants in the prior month, representing a 65 percent increase in 15 years. The World Health Organization reported in 2015 that depression is the "single largest contributor to global disability." Anxiety is ranked as the sixth. Furthermore, stress seems to be a contributing factor to a number of diseases including heart disease, depression, asthma, diabetes, and even Alzheimer's. Many common maladies can be linked to our inability to resolve, manage, or tolerate stress. The way we breathe is integral to helping us deal with stressful situations. Therefore, a daily breathing practice suddenly becomes less of a self-help approach for those seeking to improve quality of life and more like something as important to our health as brushing our teeth. We discuss breathing and its relationship to stress more in Breath and the Nervous System (page 14).

## Physical Performance

Athletes regularly use breathing techniques to enhance performance, and adaptations to breathing are the subject of much study in the field of exercise science. For example, a 2018 study on recreational runners showed improved performance efficiency (PE) in runners who train to breathe through their noses rather than through their mouths. They showed improvements in health without a loss of performance ability, even at peak levels of exercise intensity.

Professional free divers practice *voluntary prolonged apnea*—long breath holds. These athletes become desensitized to inhibited oxygen supply and the corresponding buildup of carbon dioxide. This kind of training would seem to put the athlete at an aerobic disadvantage, but instead, within certain parameters, athletes adapt, and PE improves. This technique is commonly taught to competitive swimmers and other athletes wishing to improve aerobic performance.

If you watch world-class tennis athletes play, you'll notice every strike of the ball is nearly always accompanied by a short, sharp chirp or grunt. Professional athletes know that coordinating the retention and release of the breath intensifies the power of their efforts. This technique, known as the Valsalva maneuver, is practiced by a range of athletes, from weight lifters to high jumpers.

Beyond enhancing physical performance, however, many pro athletes use focused breathing to mentally prepare for competition. Here we see that breath is used to calm nerves and clear the mind for the task at hand.

## Clarity and Focus

To improve their accuracy, the US military teaches snipers a breathing technique called "box breathing." Snipers are required to execute absolute precision in a high-stress situation with life-or-death stakes. Many of us have experience with techniques designed to help us relax in order to cope with stress. However, some situations call for the calm we associate with relaxation but the absolute clarity we associate with stress. Consider a surgeon performing a complicated procedure or the requirements of a first responder. Controlled breathing can help us become alert and focused when needed. Later, different breathing exercises can seamlessly assist our transition into a state of ease and recovery when the stress of the moment has passed.

## Sleep

If you're reading this book, chances are you were well fed and safe when you crawled into bed last night. Yet chances are also that you or someone you know has struggled with poor sleep or insomnia.

Experts believe an overactive sympathetic nervous system (discussed more on page 14) is a likely contributor to some forms of insomnia. Poor sleep interferes with the body's ability to repair itself and the immune system's ability to stave off illness. If too much stress is a contributing factor to common ailments such as poor sleep, enhancing our capacity to recognize and resolve our biological responses to stress once they are no longer needed is key. Because it addresses the nervous system directly, breath can be a powerful aid to calming us and manifesting the internal environment necessary for deep and restful sleep.

## Pain

According to a study conducted by the National Academy of Medicine, 100 million Americans suffer from chronic pain. Pain is a complex issue with a variety of potential causes, from injury to illness and even post-traumatic stress disorder (PTSD). Pain that lasts more than 12 weeks often becomes difficult to treat, and many people resign themselves to living with it indefinitely. Regardless of the causes, relaxation techniques, including breathing, have a positive effect on pain and the social-emotional consequences of dealing with the stress of chronic pain.

## Well-being

Mindfulness techniques such as yoga and meditation are at the forefront of suggested ways to manage overall stress, including the sense of disconnection and malaise that seem to be an all-too-common symptom of modern living. Regardless of age, we all suffer. All of us will eventually experience a personal crisis such as a divorce, illness, or death of a loved one. And all of us will age. How to handle these events, as well as how to bring meaning into our everyday lives, experience more joy in our relationships, and inspire well-being within ourselves are the topics of countless self-help books and wellness programs. Whether through stillness, mindfulness, expressive art, affirmation, or community service, experts commonly recommend we regularly engage in some kind of personal practice that alters our perspective.

Conscious breathing as an act of mindfulness promotes introspection and allows us to step out of the duties and responsibilities of our lives for a brief period of time in order to recalibrate and tune in to ourselves and our sense of purpose.

## Breath as Cure?

More research needs to be done into the complex relationship between breathing, stress, disease, and healing. But today you and everyone around you have free and immediate access to a tool that literally nourishes your very cells, supports your body's natural inclination to repair itself, reduces the physical and psychological implications of your complex life, and can help you cultivate well-being.

# The Importance of Carbon Dioxide

The cellular process of oxidation for cellular energy results in two waste byproducts: water ($H_2O$) and carbon dioxide ($CO_2$). Excess $CO_2$ is returned to the bloodstream and carried back to the lungs to be released from the body.

$CO_2$ is more than just waste, however. Contrary to what we may think, the body regulates our respiration, including breathing rate and volume, primarily based on our levels of $CO_2$, not our levels of oxygen. $CO_2$ also plays an important role in maintaining blood pH (pH is a measure of acidity).

Blood pH is one of the most carefully regulated systems in the human body: It will tolerate no more than a .05 deviation from pH 7.4. The renal system is the primary and most accurate gatekeeper of blood pH, but it takes about 30 minutes for the kidneys to filter all the blood in the body. If blood pH levels deviate suddenly, the effects can be devastating to organs and tissues and can lead to coma and even death. Respiration is the body's backup system and can swiftly bring pH levels back within range by adjusting $CO_2$. Faster breathing throws off excess $CO_2$. Slow breathing helps the body retain $CO_2$.

Many in alternative health communities suggest that breathing practices can be used to promote less acidity in the human body for improved health. However, barring the presence of certain diseases, severe metabolic dysfunction, or intoxication, the human body is extremely effective at spontaneously regulating pH via the respiratory system. Though breathing exercises do affect blood chemistry, any temporary deviation of pH due to the application of breathing techniques will be quickly corrected by the body's own regulatory systems.

You breathe every day but are usually unaware of it. You may now wish to consider whether you experience challenges that are related to poor breathing habits. It's possible we have individually, collectively, and across cultures underestimated the intrinsic value of conscious breathing. Pause. Take a breath. My sincere hope is that you will find some of what you need here to get past those challenges.

## What Is Breathing, and Why Do We Do It?

The human body is made up of around 37.2 trillion cells, all of which need oxygen to survive. Put most simply, breathing is the act of pulling air into the body in order to bring in $O_2$, then letting it out to relieve the body of $CO_2$. A coordinated effort is made by a number of muscles, including the diaphragm, intercostal muscles, and various support muscles, to shape the thoracic cavity (the area inside the ribs) so that air is pulled into our lungs. Corresponding muscles, along with the elastic properties of the affected tissues, assist air back out. This cycle happens, mostly unconsciously, around 12 times a minute.

Impressively, the surface area inside our lungs is comparable to the surface area of a tennis court. The primary goal when taking a breath is to expose an appropriate amount of that surface area to the air breathed in. Our bodies continuously adjust breath volume and frequency in order to adapt to the variable needs of our cells for fuel. Like heartbeat and digestion, breathing is regulated by the autonomic nervous system (ANS), which is responsible for bodily functions that do not require conscious direction. Notably, breathing is the only autonomic function in the body that we can also consciously direct.

# Physical Structures Related to Breathing

**Nose:** Breath enters the body through the nostrils, which are lined with tiny hairs to filter the air on its way in.

**Turbinates:** Shell-shaped networks of bone and fleshy, moist tissues line the nasal passages and help regulate the temperature and humidity of incoming air. Mucus further cleans the air before it continues into the lungs. Turbinate tissue is erectile, alternately swelling and constricting. When turbinate swelling congests one nasal passage, the turbinate tissue in the other passage constricts. This is a natural, rhythmic process that happens several times a day and does not affect overall airflow in a healthy person.

**Epiglottis:** This flap of tissue at the base of the tongue closes the airway when we swallow.

**Glottis:** The area of the throat that houses the vocal cords changes shape to regulate the flow of air as it passes through. The space the air passes through is referred to as the glottis.

**Airways:** The trachea, bronchi, and bronchioli transport air into the lungs. The trachea is commonly referred to as the "windpipe." It bifurcates into two sets of bronchi; each then further branches into smaller bronchioli that terminate at small sacs called alveoli. These passages are moistened with mucus, which helps trap dust and particulates and assists these contaminants back out of the airways before they reach the alveoli.

**Lungs:** We have two lungs, each consisting of bronchi, bronchioli, and alveoli. In most of us, the lung on the left has two distinct lobes, and the lung on the right has three. It is thought the left lung is smaller to allow space in the thorax for the heart.

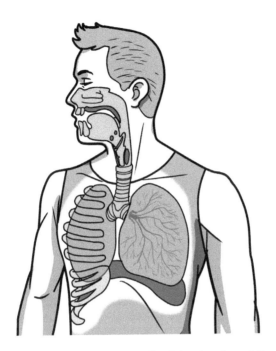

**Alveoli:** Tiny inflatable sacs are the final destination of the air that enters the lungs. The thin membranous surface of the alveoli walls is where blood is exposed to oxygen. Oxygen and carbon dioxide are exchanged here through the process of diffusion.

**Thorax:** The breastbone (sternum), the ribs (costae), and the 12 vertebrae to which the ribs attach (thoracic spine) join to form the thorax, the cage-like structure that protects our heart and lungs. The act of breathing affects the volume of the thoracic cavity, causing air to rush into or out of the lungs.

**Diaphragm:** When at rest this large parachute-shaped muscle (attached to the lowest six ribs, the lower part of the sternum, and the lumbar spine) domes high into the thorax. It flattens downward during inhalation, and returns to its domed shape during exhalation.

# 3-MINUTE BASELINE

This exercise will help you establish your baseline, which you can use later to assess progress. You will need:

» A timer

» A place to record your results

» A comfortable place to sit

Find a comfortable, quiet place to sit. The only requirement for your seated posture is that you sit up straight so that your breathing is uninhibited. It is not necessary to sit on the floor.

Set your timer for 3 minutes. Close your eyes and begin to count your breaths. When the timer alerts you that 3 minutes have passed, make a mental note of the number of breaths you took. Continue to sit for another minute or so and take notice of *how you feel*. Be careful not to impose ideas about how you *think* you should feel. Be honest. This is important.

# Record Your Observations

Record today's date and roughly how many breaths you took in three minutes. As you develop your breathing, you will naturally start to take fewer breaths during this exercise. A word of warning, however: If you approach the exercise with impatience, insisting on fewer breaths rather than letting it happen naturally, you will quickly find yourself short of breath and anxious. Breathing is not a competition. You are breathing to feel better, not to prove something to yourself or anyone else. We will revisit your baseline at the end of each week so you can track your progress.

Jot down anything else that you noticed during the exercise. If you found your mind wandering, write that down. If you found yourself noticing any part of your physical body, record that. Nothing is off limits. Jot down any insights that came to you—for example, "Hmmm, I never noticed before how tense my shoulders are" or "I was feeling so agitated during this. I wonder if it had to do with that extra cup of coffee I drank this morning." Your insights are your subconscious becoming conscious.

# Breath and the Nervous System

Most of us breathe every day without any real trouble. We may be conscious of our breath only when we exert ourselves or yawn or if we for some reason have our air supply cut off. At the same time, we may have a host of issues that, though we don't attribute them to poor breathing habits, can be addressed by improving how we breathe. As mentioned earlier, many of the things that trouble us have stress as an underlying factor. Let's take a closer look at the nervous system and how unconscious use of the breath can do us a disservice, whereas breathing consciously can be a game changer for our health.

## The Autonomic Nervous System (ANS)

The ANS is responsible for the functions of your body that you do not control consciously, including breathing, heart rate, and digestion. Two complementary branches work in opposition to help us maintain homeostasis. The *sympathetic nervous system* (SNS) is considered an accelerator and is generally associated with functions requiring quick responses. The *parasympathetic nervous system* (PNS) can be seen as a decelerator and is associated with functions that do not require immediate action. Both systems profoundly influence and can be influenced by the breath.

## Fight or Flight

The SNS is designed to keep us alive. Under the threat of harm, the SNS activates, *increasing* heart rate, blood pressure, and breathing. During this process the "higher" brain takes a little vacation, and the prehistoric "survival" brain takes over. When the SNS is activated, blood is diverted from less critical organs to the skeletal muscles, which may require extra energy to either move us to safety or fend off danger. The emotions associated with SNS activation are primarily fear, anger, mistrust, and excitement. The SNS is associated with *rapid chest breathing.*

## Rest, Play, Love

The PNS has an inverse relationship to the SNS. The PNS conserves energy by *decreasing* heart rate, blood pressure, and breathing when we are at rest. Blood flow is diverted from skeletal muscles to organs such as those responsible for digestion. Some primary emotions associated with the PNS are contentment, gratitude, trust, and joy. *Full, slow breaths* are natural to the PNS.

## Insights from Asthma

*Stress, an SNS experience, is a well-known contributor to asthmatic symptoms. Clinicians now prescribe breath awareness and controlled breathing to help patients identify the early warning signs of an attack and stave off acute episodes.*

## Breathing Habits

We should consider how our personal breathing style plays a role in influencing the biological mechanisms associated with the ANS. For example, poor breathing habits might include shallow chest breathing due to reasons other than anxiety, such as poor posture, sedentary lifestyle, or a simple lack of awareness. Chest breathing is what your body does to help you cope with fear. Just as we may use slower, fuller breathing to calm the SNS, shallow chest breathing can stimulate the SNS and the biological changes that go with it, including rapid heart rate, release of stress hormones, and mental vigilance.

Usually, mortal threat is not the cause of our stress. Modern stress has more to do with overwork and overwhelm. Modern humans experience a tendency to prioritize things we *think* will make us happy, such as making more money at a stressful job, instead of things that actually make us happy, such as spending more time with our loved ones, building community, or engaging in service. When we are stressed as a result of these choices, the SNS is online. Though we can't control where our body sends our blood or how fast our heart beats, we do have direct control over how we breathe.

### Slow It Down

"Slow down, breathe." Instinctively we know that after being startled, we can assist the recovery process by taking deeper, longer breaths. If the things that cause us distress and disease are exacerbated by stress, finding healthy ways to resolve stress makes sense. We know breathing can help us when we're in the middle of a crisis, but let's take this line of thinking a step further.

What might the implications be of getting ahead of stress by integrating healthy, PNS-supportive breathing exercises into our daily lives *before* we're in a crisis? Not only might we better manage chronic or low-level stress before it becomes a health problem, we might also wind up with better-developed strategies for handling the more intense moments that are an inevitable part of living active, engaged lives.

## Breathing Techniques: How to Choose

A quick Internet search yields hundreds of websites describing varied breathing practices. Yoga and other ancient philosophical and religious traditions offer techniques that differ slightly from school to school. Breathing exercises come to us through medical sources for specific conditions, such as asthma or COPD. Organizations devoted to public health, such as The American Institute of Stress, offer breathing recommendations, and a plethora of self-help gurus and athletic-performance aficionados promote trademarked breathing exercises and systems for improved health. Adding to the confusion, scientific research on the effects of breathing is plentiful and promising, but the quality of studies varies, as do the breathing techniques used and the resulting recommendations. All this information can make it difficult to determine which practices might be useful to integrate into our lives.

Most breathing exercises, regardless of their origins, fall into the eight following types:

## Breath Awareness

Probably the most straightforward and accessible practice, breath awareness is the act of simply paying attention to our breathing. This brings the unconscious act of breathing into conscious awareness. Taking time to notice our breathing often leads to introspection and also *interoception* (the ability to feel sensation inside the body).

## Belly Breathing

Sometimes referred to as "diaphragmatic breathing," belly breathing focuses effort on mobilizing the diaphragm, the dome-shaped muscle between the thoracic and abdominal cavities. During its first phase of contraction, the diaphragm increases the volume of the lungs by flattening and descending toward the abdomen. During inhalation, the downward movement displaces the abdominal organs, and the abdomen distends. The second phase of diaphragmatic contraction lifts and separates the lowest ribs, contributing to Rib Cage Breathing (see next section). Belly breathing is efficient when we are at rest.

## Rib Cage Breathing

Sometimes referred to as "chest breathing" or "costal breathing," rib cage breathing refers to the mobilization of the rib cage due to the second phase of diaphragmatic contraction (see Belly Breathing), along with the participation of skeletal muscles in order to increase and decrease thoracic volume. We naturally engage in costal breathing when we are exerting ourselves, such as during intense physical exercise.

## Resistance Breathing

Applying resistance to the breath as it moves into and out of the body is a technique designed to strengthen the respiratory and cardiovascular muscles. Though they have other applications, special branded devices such as Expand-a-Lung® and PowerLung® exist to provide artificial resistance. They are commonly promoted to people with ailments such as COPD and asthma and to athletes, singers, and musicians who play wind instruments. Resistance can be created naturally at the mouth by pursing the lips or curling the tongue or at the throat by narrowing the aperture of the glottis (such as when we talk, whisper, or sing). Modern postural yoga practitioners commonly employ resistance breathing, which generates a soft snoring sound, during postural practice. Controlling the pace of breathing becomes easier with this technique, as the stream of air is regulated where the breath enters and leaves the body as opposed to the coordinated control of larger muscle groups, such as the intercostal muscles and the diaphragm.

## The Breath Wave and Circular Breathing

Known as *anulom valom* in Sanskrit, circular breathing is considered the foundation of yoga pranayama. It encourages a coordinated effort of the musculoskeletal structures that come into motion when we breathe in order to use full lung capacity. At the start of inhalation, the practitioner actively distends the abdominal muscles to support diaphragmatic activation. As inhalation continues, there is an ascending expansion of the rib cage sequentially from the lower ribs to the highest ribs. During exhalation the practitioner encourages a descending contraction of the rib cage from the higher ribs to the lowest ribs. Toward the end of exhalation the abdominal muscles pull in, supporting the upward movement of the diaphragm.

## Fast Breathing

We inherit two common fast-breathing techniques from yoga traditions. The breath of fire (*kapalabhati*) focuses on exhalation and encourages a rapid and continuous contraction and release of the abdominal muscles to expel and recover short puffs of air. This technique relies on the elasticity of the tissues after exhalation for the return of air into the lungs. Bellows breathing (*bhastrika*) is a more aggressive diaphragmatic technique that employs a rapid, forceful exhalation *and* inhalation. Both fast-breathing techniques encourage a state of hyperventilation, temporarily reducing $CO_2$ in the bloodstream and increasing the ratio of oxygen comparatively.

## Alternate Nostril Breathing

Borrowed from age-old yoga traditions, alternate nostril breathing (*nadi shodhana*) is a technique in which the practitioner alternately closes or blocks one nostril for a complete breath cycle. Traditional yoga energy theory references two central energy channels (*nadis*) that are thought to be stimulated by variations of this breathing technique. Alternate nostril breathing is associated with SNS activation, particularly during inhalation when breathing through the right nostril, and

## Through the Nose, Not the Mouth

In this book we sometimes use mouth breathing as a temporary learning tool. In healthy individuals, breathing through the mouth is not a problem. The body naturally opts for mouth breathing when there is a need to shift from breathing through the nose in favor of a more efficient way to get oxygen to the lungs, such as when exercising or when congested due to a cold or sinus infection.

Please note that breathing habits that incorporate chronic mouth breathing, a state in which one habitually breathes both in and out through the mouth, can have long-term health effects, including snoring, sleep apnea, increased allergies, dry mouth, and bad breath. People who suffer from frequent sinus infections, chronic allergies, or asthma sometimes continue mouth breathing even between bouts of congestion, simply from habit. Chronic overbreathing, a condition where one breathes through the mouth as if short of breath, can interfere with $O_2$:$CO_2$ ratios in the blood.

There are significant benefits to breathing through the nose. The nasal passages warm, humidify, clean, and slow incoming air, preparing it for the lungs. In addition, paranasal sinuses—air-filled cavities within the bones of the skull located above, below, and between the eyes—produce nitrous oxide (NO) and continuously release the gas into the nasal passages. NO has antibacterial, antiviral, antiparasitic, and antifungal properties. Its presence helps protect the body from outside invaders and also dilates blood vessels, contributing to improved transport and absorption of oxygen.

PNS activation, particularly during exhalation when breathing through the left nostril. Studies on brain wave patterns also suggest a relationship between the right and left nostrils and corresponding left and right brain hemisphere activity.

### Timing and Suspending the Breath

A counting structure that regulates the pace of breathing is referred to as a *timing*. A variety of breath timings along with breath holds, or suspensions, are common to Eastern breathing systems including yoga. Celebrity doctor and holistic medical proponent Andrew Weil popularized the 4:7:8 breath for its relaxing properties and as an aid to sleep. In this technique the breath is inhaled for 4 counts, held for 7 counts, then exhaled for 8 counts (we will practice the 4:7:8 breath in week 3).

A timing helps us adjust the duration of any given part of the breath cycle relative to another. Suspending breathing, or holding the breath, supports PNS activation, perhaps by encouraging the body to redirect blood flow away from skeletal muscles and toward vital organs as oxygen levels deplete. Excessive holding of the breath can be dangerous and in some cases may exacerbate anxiety, so our application of these techniques will be selective and gentle.

## Breathing-Related Health Problems

If your interest in Breathwork comes as a result of a physical issue like COPD, asthma, or allergies, you will likely be more interested in week 1 (see page 67), which directly addresses the physiological aspects of better breathing and provides practices that can benefit these challenges. I invite you to revisit that chapter as often as needed.

Do continue on with weeks 2 and 3, however. As mentioned, some physiological health problems are related to how we manage stress, which we address in week 2. In week 3 we remember that one of our overall goals of improving our breathing is enhanced well-being. Staying with the program for the full three weeks will support you in establishing an ongoing breathing practice. This is probably the single most important factor to your potential success.

As you become proficient at Breathwork, I fully expect you to notice improvements in your physical health. At the same time, it is important to remember that even though breathing is a natural approach to healing, many medical conditions require medical intervention. Breathing practices should not be substituted, at least initially, for treatments prescribed by your doctor or caregiver without their consent. Often the best approach for treating disease is a coordinated effort between you and your medical caregiver. You must take full responsibility for supporting your body in its ability to heal itself by making informed lifestyle choices that include adequate exercise, excellent nutrition, and reduced stress. Though a breathing practice should absolutely be an integral part of your healthy lifestyle, use it *with* and not instead of your doctor's recommendations.

## Establishing Your Practice

It is said that whatever is worth doing at all is worth doing well. If you do not have prior experience with breathing practices, give yourself both time and patience to fully engage with the learning curve. Certain exercises won't feel natural to you. At times you will question your efforts. There will be moments when you won't know if you're doing it right.

When you step into any new endeavor, you have to allow for the discomfort of being a beginner. The first hurdle to setting up a regular breathing practice may be quite simply the uneasiness of trying something new. Over time, your familiarity with these practices will grow, and eventually you will become an expert. Remember, every expert was once a beginner.

When you are a beginner, repetition offers the experience necessary to explore and integrate what you learn. Repetition shines a light on your strengths and your challenges. With this information you can determine where to direct your efforts in order to improve. If you continue with Breathwork beyond this program, at a certain point you will know the techniques well enough, because you have done them so many times, that you will be able to make your own evaluations of them and tailor them to your needs.

Consistency is also important. Practicing regularly and for a sustained period of time will help you enjoy better results from your efforts. When you practice regularly, you develop a deeper awareness of your personal habits and styles. Furthermore, the consistency of your practice serves as a backdrop for all that is ever changing in your energy, mood, and effort, helping you to better know and understand yourself in relationship to all that is moving and changing around you.

## Journal

This might be a nice time to establish a practice journal. Whether you use a computer, pen and paper, or the voice recorder on your phone, consider taking some notes or jotting down some thoughts about the challenges and rewards of establishing a practice. The following are some questions to answer:

## Commitment: Your Will

In order for Breathwork to work, practice needs to be a priority, and you will need to commit. This is a three-week complete breathing program, and we will be breathing intentionally every day. Are you ready to commit to a regular daily practice?

## Intentions: Your Why

By now you probably have some ideas about why you are interested in Breathwork. What are your specific goals? Are they realistic? Are you hopeful? Skeptical? Record your *why*. Be as specific as possible. By the way, you can have more than one *why*!

## Make Time: Your When

It's important to make time in your schedule to practice. To move forward with this program, you will need to put aside less than 30 minutes per day. In general, we practice twice daily: 10 minutes in the morning and 10 to 20 minutes in the evening. Think about how you will need to adjust your current routine to accommodate this, and record in your journal your strategy to make time for daily practice for 21 days in a row. Pull out your planner and look for any conflicts that might derail you. Be very thoughtful about this. Making time can be one of the biggest challenges to establishing a regular practice.

## Make Space: Your Where

Breathing practice doesn't need special equipment or a dedicated space. You just need enough space in which to lie down—at home, in your office, outside, anywhere you're comfortable. You don't always need privacy, just a few moments of quiet. In all likelihood, when you practice will determine where you practice, or the other way around. Is there anything you need to do to make space?

## Gather Resources: Your Support

You don't need special clothes or gear to practice breathing, though it helps to be comfortable. Gather the following supplies for your morning and evening practices:

» Two or three similar size thin blankets

» Straight-backed chair, such as a dining chair

» Yoga strap (available at almost any department store) or other fully adjustable belt

» Notebook, journal, or laptop to record progress but also insights, ideas, memories, and emotions

> *Tell a friend! Someone you love or trust can be an excellent resource. Sometimes telling another of our intentions helps us follow through. Consider reaching out to this person when you need encouragement, or ask them to check in with you toward the end of each week to give you kudos and lend support.*

## Breathing Your Way to Better Health

Our goal is to practice twice a day for 21 days straight. Practicing daily without a break offers you an immersive opportunity to reach a level of competency and comfort in order to feel ready to carry the practice into your routine moving forward.

You may start your practice on any day of the week. If you do shift work or have an alternative schedule, feel free to adapt your start day or time accordingly. Why 21 days? Three weeks of practice is doable. One month may be too much to ask; two weeks isn't enough time to establish a good routine. The time line I've detailed here is needed to introduce the concepts and practices I believe are most useful and that you'll want to carry forward.

The following is a breakdown of the general focus of the program, week by week.

## Week 1: Cultivating Integration

Our practice in week 1 focuses on the physical aspects of Breathwork. By turning the mind's attention toward the physical body, we support mind-body integration, reinforcing the bridge between our physical selves and our thoughts, ideas, and emotions. During this period you will learn three foundational breathing techniques that you will refine in weeks 2 and 3: belly breathing, rib cage breathing, and resistance breathing.

## Week 2: Cultivating Awareness

We turn our attention in week 2 toward using the breath to enhance awareness of our emotional and intellectual selves. Awareness is key to understanding how to use Breathwork to address issues such as anxiety, insomnia, and depression. After seven days, the practice routine will be starting to feel familiar, and you will begin to refine your technique and build in variations. You will start to identify the breathing practices you favor and that come easily to you, as well as those which are more challenging. This week, we explore variations of the three foundational techniques from week 1 and add circular breathing and timings to your repertoire.

## Week 3: Cultivating Connection

In our final week, we explore how Breathwork can support us in our overall well-being. This week we add a layer of intentionality and play with the ways in which our breathing can enhance our senses of belonging, purpose, and presence. Techniques will encourage connection through breathing to the deeper aspects of our selves, to others, and to our environment. By the end of week 3 you will have experience with alternate nostril breathing and suspending your breath, and you will leave our 21-day program with a short menu of complete breathing practices to take with you.

## Optional Afternoon Practices: Pausing and Remembering

An afternoon practice—a breath break—can serve as a touchstone during a busy day. In a few minutes you can enjoy an afternoon reset with a quick body scan or a simple breathing practice that will leave you feeling steady and reenergized.

In weeks 2 and 3 I have included two special practices that would serve nicely as afternoon additions to your daily routine. However, any Breathwork exercise may be brought into the middle part of your day.

## Breathwork and Beyond

The practices presented in this book provide a solid foundation for incorporating Breathwork toward our shared goal of improved health and enhanced well-being. If you stick with the program, not only will you come out of these 21 days with better breathing habits and an improved understanding of the positive benefits of conscious breathing, you will also emerge physically healthier, emotionally renewed, and newly inspired.

## Chapter Two

# Foundations

For Breathwork to be effective, you will want to develop a handful of foundational habits and techniques to take forward into the weeks ahead. When we approach practice thoughtfully and with intention, we create an optimal environment for success. This chapter offers some practical tips and tools, and includes some additional information and considerations for our time together.

# Best Practices

You can use this chapter as a reference—come back to it at any time during this program as questions arise. Later in this chapter I have included instructions for two preparatory practices that you will incorporate daily as part of your morning and evening exercises. For some of the exercises and meditations, you will find links to audio recordings or video tutorials on my website, to help establish familiarity with the techniques.

## The Importance of Staying Relaxed

First and foremost, when we practice breathing we must practice with ease. It is important to stay relaxed. The body scan meditation (see page 52) helps us develop awareness of the physical tension we habitually hold in our bodies. When we practice with tension we reinforce it, and it is unlikely to resolve. In order to resolve tension, first we must become aware of it. Once we're aware, we can learn to release it and move forward in our practice (and our lives) without it. I will be reminding you throughout to regularly check for and release tension when you find it.

If you think about it, it takes effort to hold tension in your body. This effort requires energy that could be directed toward something else. If you had extra energy, what would you do with it?

## Timing Your Practice

Timing your practice can help you stick with a given practice for a little longer than you would naturally, allowing you to gradually increase your comfort level with the exercise. Or it can keep you from losing track of time so, for example, your practice doesn't cause you to be late for work.

For our daily sessions, I have opted to limit most of the exercises to three to five minutes for two reasons: First, if you are new to seated practice, you will start to feel uncomfortable after about three minutes. If you're uncomfortable, you'll be less likely to continue with Breathwork. Second, finding time for daily practice can be a challenge. If practices are short, you may be more likely to fit them into your schedule.

Feel free to adjust the length of time to suit your disposition. A word of warning, though: Your perception of your busy life and your need for efficiency could cause you to rush your practice, which means you could miss out on its benefits. What I offer here should be considered the minimum—a place to start when you are just beginning.

When you do notice benefits or even fall in love with some of the exercises, you may intuitively begin to desire more practice time. Let it be this desire that guides you into longer practice periods rather than a preconceived notion of how long you should spend with Breathwork.

To precisely time your Breathwork, use the built-in stopwatch app on your smartphone. Choose an alert that is calming, such, music or a meditative gong. This way, the timer can play its tune without startling you, and you will not need to stop your breathing to turn off the alarm right away. There is a wonderful free app called Insight Timer that works well for meditation.

## Transitions

During seated practice our bodies can become stagnant. Sometimes our legs fall asleep, or we start to feel pain from sitting in one position for too long. Traditional schools of meditation teach that we should dissociate from the body by observing these sensations without responding to them. In these schools, transcending physical discomfort is seen as a way of transcending the body itself, in the service of another ideal. Though that may be appropriate for certain kinds of spiritual practices, our purpose here is different. We wish to develop a synergistic relationship with our bodies for the sake of improved health. Overstressing your body by ignoring the messages it has for you can lead to pain, frustration, and even injury.

Like a nurturing caregiver, listen to the questions your body is asking of you. Honor discomfort with attention and gentle movements when necessary. As we work toward combining techniques, which results in longer practices, I will encourage you to stretch your legs and adjust your body during transitions between exercises. Keeping the body focused yet relaxed during practice is a skill worth developing, but whenever you need to change positions or gently stretch, do so.

## Repetition

As we work through our 21 days together, we will repeat skills regularly, building in nuance and adding variations every day. Because we are building skills, these weeks of practice will include much more variation than your ongoing practice should.

After week 3, I encourage you to either repeat this program from beginning to end to solidify your knowledge, or settle into the simple, repetitive routines I suggest in week 3. If you do choose a more repetitive practice, revisiting the full program periodically will refresh you in the basics and reacquaint you with some of the exercises you initially opted not to include in your ongoing practice.

## Tuning In

After each practice, you will be invited to briefly tune in to how you feel. This is an important component of Breathwork. The goal by the end of the program is for you to be familiar with the exercises in this book. In the absence of a teacher, your experience with how the exercises make you feel and how they affect you in the hours after practice will be integral to deciding which exercises to work with moving forward and which to leave out of your practice for now.

For example, if you identify as a type A person, you may notice you do not need the stimulating breath of fire and may opt instead to stick with belly breathing in the morning. You will know what works for you by becoming an expert in tuning in. None of us feels the same every day, of course, but you will start to observe some patterns and learn which breathing exercises work best for you.

## Your Practice Journal

As mentioned, it is helpful to keep a practice journal. You'll keep a weekly log of your progress, so you can see how Breathwork is affecting you. I encourage you to journal after each practice, even if you record only a sentence or two. This is a place to jot down the thoughts, ideas, insights, memories, and observations that occur as a result of your work. With this kind of reflection you may more easily start to see a connection between Breathwork and how it is benefitting your everyday life.

If you are not inclined to journal, your smartphone has a voice recorder. Pull it out and record a few thoughts on your way to work or in the evening as you prepare a meal or get ready for bed.

Here is an example of a short journal entry:

*February 20. 7:30 a.m. Breath Prep Stretch and Release + Alternate Nostril Breathing. 10 minutes. Feeling relaxed but was thinking a lot about work.*

## Pacing Yourself

My goal is to help you establish a daily practice that you *want* to keep coming back to—one that is simple and accessible and provides immediate benefits. We all learn at different rates and come to the practice with different levels of experience. As you work through the Breathwork

### Literally, breath is movement

If we inhibit movement with poor posture or a sedentary lifestyle, we inherently inhibit our breathing. The first part of recovery is releasing tension to allow for motion. The second is to encourage the intelligent and natural integration of the different organs and muscles responsible for the movements of respiration.

program, revisit each week or repeat days as necessary. At the same time, resist the urge to skip certain exercises or rush ahead. The daily exercises build upon each other, and the vocabulary you establish as you work forward each day is foundational to your future success. If you don't make it through all of the practices in 21 days because you have repeated practice days, that is not a problem! Celebrate practicing 21 days in a row, then continue with the program until you finish.

## Potential Complications

If you have health-related problems or are taking prescription medications, please consult your caregiver before beginning Breathwork. Barring medical conditions that may restrict you from practicing, occasionally minor physical barriers will come up.

**Congestion:** Your nose may become congested due to a cold or allergies. In this case, many of the exercises will be impossible. If the nose is partially congested, fast-breathing techniques can sometimes stimulate the erectile tissue in the inflamed nasal passages to contract, which can free the nostrils for practice. However, if you are congested and breathing is restricted, you may opt to do some of the exercises through the mouth or rest and wait for the sinuses to clear.

**Anxiety:** If you are feeling anxious, some of the exercises may seem frightening, as if they will leave you feeling too vulnerable. Tension in the throat, belly, or jaw—common side effects of anxiety—may restrict your access to some of the exercises. It is okay to continue with your breathing practice, although when anxiety is troubling you or seems to be interfering with your practice, stick with the simplest exercises from week 1 and the calming evening exercises from weeks 1 and 2. Slow, smooth belly breathing is your go-to during periods of more acute anxiety.

**Asthma:** Some students with asthma report that in the beginning, the breathing exercises feel unsettling. Controlling one's breathing highlights the possibility that one could potentially lose control of one's breathing. Resistance breathing in particular can be reminiscent of the restriction people with asthma experience during an episode. Most students report that after they become accustomed to Breathwork, they find the opposite is true. They come to feel empowered by new tools to help them manage their condition. If you have asthma, consult your doctor before beginning Breathwork. Then go slowly and allow yourself all the time you need to acclimate to the exercises.

# *Practice Basics*

In order to begin Breathwork, you will need to be familiar with the following postures and gentle stretches, as well as the short guided meditation presented below. We will regularly incorporate these practices throughout. You probably feel eager to get started and may wonder if it's really necessary to include these steps. Breathwork will be most effective in combination with these simple foundational techniques.

# SITTING FOR PRACTICE

Many of our practices take place while we are seated. While we commonly think of seated practice as sitting cross-legged on the floor, this posture can be problematic for some, as the knees and hips and can get uncomfortable quickly. Breathwork (and meditation) can be done in any position. You may sit at your desk, in your car, or, better yet, outside—perhaps under a tree or on a park bench. The only requirement is that you sit up straight. If you slouch, your posture will interfere with your ability to breathe.

Renowned meditation teacher and Sanskrit scholar Lorin Roche, PhD, provides a wonderful observation about choosing a seated posture. He reminds practitioners that the only thing we gain when we move from a chair to the floor is that sitting on the floor "looks cooler!"

*Steps*

**1.** Choose a comfortable place to sit, either in a chair or on the floor. Rest your hands in your lap and completely relax them. Relax your face, and relax your jaw.

**2.** Bring your awareness to the bones at the base of your pelvis. Press down through the base of your pelvis and lengthen your spine upward, toward the ceiling.

**3.** As you lift your spine tall, allow your shoulders to release down, away from your ears. You are now in an optimal position for breathing. Work to maintain this posture for the duration of your seated practice.

---

**Tip:** *When sitting in a chair, sit forward toward the front of the chair, so both feet rest comfortably on the floor. Sit tall and straight, but without rigidity. If you choose to sit on the floor, consider elevating your pelvis several inches by sitting on a firm surface. In figure 2.1, the practitioner is sitting on a stack of neatly folded blankets, but a firm cushion or even a stack of books will work. It's fine to lean up against a wall as long as you are not reclining.*

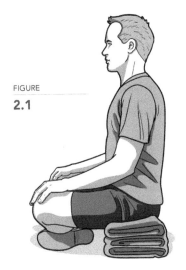

FIGURE

**2.1**

# RECLINED RESTING POSE

After certain practices you will be encouraged to take a reclined rest as in figure 2.2.

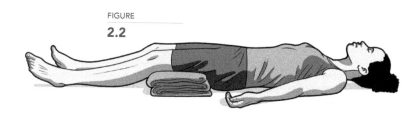

FIGURE
**2.2**

Note that the arms are away from the body, not quite straight out to the sides, but almost. This promotes expansiveness across the chest. It is fine to put a low support, such as a folded blanket, underneath the head, but it should be no more than one or two inches high. A common mistake is to use a thick pillow, which causes the head to tilt. The neck should remain in a neutral position.

## Steps

**1.** Find a quiet place to lie down. Lie on the floor, rather than on a soft surface such as a couch or bed.

**2.** Separate your feet so they are roughly hip-distance apart and take your arms away from your body with the palms facing up. Arrange your shoulder blades on the floor behind you so that they are away from your ears.

**3.** Allow your limbs to become heavy, and the weight of your pelvis, rib cage, shoulders, and head to surrender into the floor behind you.

**4.** Completely relax your hands and your feet. Completely relax your jaw. Relax your forehead, brow, and all the tiny muscles around your eyes. Relax your whole body and settle in for a few minutes of rest.

---

**Tip:** *For some, lying flat on the floor is uncomfortable for the lower back. In this case, a stack or roll of two to four blankets placed under the thighs, as shown in figure 2.2, will usually relieve any tenderness. If there is pain elsewhere in the body, choose another resting pose that works for you.*

## *Opening the Chest*
# RECLINED POSTURE

Occasionally, we will rest in a position designed to open and expand the front rib cage and chest. The reclined chest opener moves the ribs into a lifted position. This position directly contradicts the habitual slouching many of us are prone to and helps us improve or maintain the rib cage flexibility we need for healthy breathing. You will need 2 to 4 blankets to be comfortable in this pose. Here is how to set it up:

## *Steps*

**1.** Fold 2 blankets each into a rectangle about the size of a large serving tray (figure 2.3).

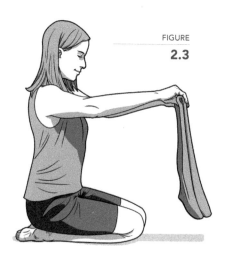

FIGURE
**2.3**

**2.** Fold the first rectangle into thirds lengthwise and accordion style (figure 2.4). Fold the second rectangle in half lengthwise. Smooth out any wrinkles or lumps.

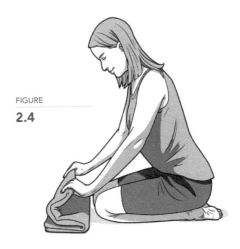

FIGURE
**2.4**

**3.** Sit on the floor, and lay the first blanket lengthwise behind you. Keep the second within reach. You may or may not need it.

**4.** Lie back on the blanket, resting the soles of your feet on the floor, with your knees up. Note that your pelvis is on the floor, not on the blanket, and the blanket is supporting both your low back and your head. If it feels comfortable to extend your legs, you may.

**5.** If your head falls back, your airway may become restricted. Lay the second blanket across the first. This blanket may serve as a slight lift for your head and may be adjusted for thickness as needed. However, the neck should remain in a neutral position (figure 2.5).

FIGURE
**2.5**

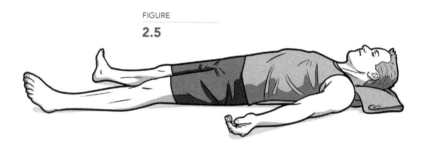

**6.** Move your arms away from your body, not quite straight out to the sides but almost. Move your shoulders down and away from your ears.

**Tip:** *If the low back is tender, place a stack or roll of 2 to 4 blankets under the thighs, as discussed in the Reclined Resting Pose (figure 2.2). The reclined chest opener may feel too intense for some. If you are at all uncomfortable, revert to the reclined resting pose. On the other hand, some prefer to stack a second folded blanket on top of the first, to further elevate the rib cage.*

# STRETCH AND RESET SEQUENCE

**Total time: 3 to 5 minutes**

We will start each morning practice with the following simple stretches. This sequence helps release tension, relieve back pain, and open the chest in preparation for Breathwork.

## Alternate Knee to Chest

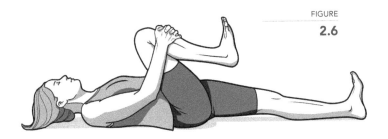

FIGURE
**2.6**

Lie down on your back and hug your knees to your chest. Bring some awareness to your breathing.

» Interlace your fingers around your right knee and straighten your left leg along the floor (figure 2.6).

» Hold for 3 to 5 breaths.

» Repeat on the other side.

## Reclined Twist

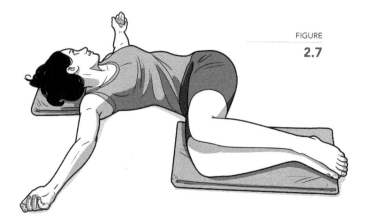

FIGURE

**2.7**

**1.** Bring both knees into your chest.

**2.** Let your knees and feet fall to the right of your torso, so your pelvis turns to the right and your spine twists (figure 2.7).

**3.** Open your left arm out to the side and turn the palm of your left hand to face up. Move both shoulders down and away from your ears.

**4.** Take 3 to 5 long, full breaths.

**5.** While exhaling, bring both knees back to center and draw them in toward your chest.

**6.** Repeat on the other side.

---

**Tip:** *If the opposite shoulder hovers above the ground, or if the knees do not release to the floor without straining, slide a folded blanket or cushion underneath your thighs to support the legs. Put enough support under the thighs (at least 4-6 inches) so the opposite shoulder blade can rest on the floor, as in figure 2.7. Some people prefer to put the blanket or cushion between the knees instead of underneath the legs.*

# Gentle Bridge

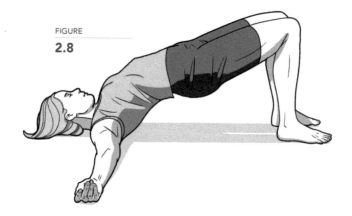

FIGURE
**2.8**

**1.** Lie on your back with the soles of your feet on the floor and your knees up. Separate your feet hip distance apart or slightly wider.

**2.** Bring your arms out to the sides and let them rest on the floor. If this causes pain in the shoulders, simply lower the arms until the shoulders don't hurt.

**3.** Move your shoulders down and away from your ears. You may need to wiggle around a little in order to adjust your shoulder blades toward your heels.

**4.** Press down into your feet and lift your hips a few inches. In this posture, the goal is not to take the hips up toward the ceiling as far as they will go, but rather to lift them just enough to bring the weight of the body onto the bulky muscles of the upper back (figure 2.8).

**5.** Play with shifting your weight from side to side, and explore putting gentle pressure on the muscles of your upper back, as if you were using the floor to give your upper back a massage. Relax your jaw.

**6.** Ease the pelvis back down to the floor.

**7.** Hug your knees back into your chest.

---

**Tip:** *If you have problems with your eyes, such as glaucoma or retinal eye disorders, or if you have had eye surgery in the last 8 weeks, skip this pose.*

# Low Cobra

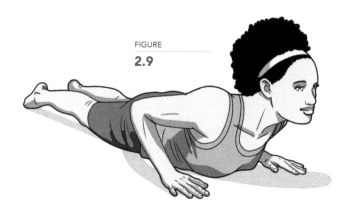

FIGURE
**2.9**

**1.** Roll onto your belly. Place your hands on either side of your rib cage, as if you were going to do a push-up.

**2.** Firm your belly in toward your spine and lift your head and chest off the floor. Take 2 or 3 breaths (figure 2.9).

**3.** Release and rest.

**4.** Repeat. Experiment with turning the head gently from side to side. Look up. Look down. Look around the room and allow your eyes to pause on landmarks around you. This process is called "orienting" and can help calm an overactive SNS.

**5.** Release the chest back down to the floor.

**6.** Repeat steps 4 and 5.

---

**Tip:** *In this position, make an effort to keep your shoulders down and away from your ears. You may find you have to adjust the position of your hands in order to press the chest up without the shoulders lifting. If you press up too high, your lower back may start to hurt. Simply do less.*

*When you strain, you are bypassing the "reset" and charging head on into fight or flight mode. You will know you are straining if you have pain, your breathing becomes labored, or you find yourself holding your breath.*

# Reclined Squat

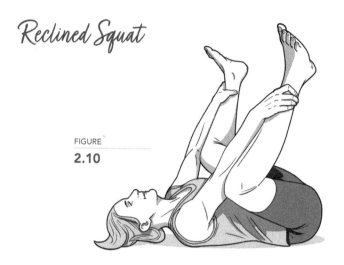

FIGURE
**2.10**

**1.** Slowly roll back onto your back and bring your knees in toward your chest.

**2.** Reach down for your big toes. With the palms of your hands facing each other, hold on to your big toes with your index and second fingers.

**3.** Part your thighs and gently draw them down toward the floor on either side of your rib cage. Keep the thighs in toward the sides of your ribs and turn the soles of your feet to face the ceiling.

**4.** Hold for 5 to 7 breaths. Release your knees back to your chest.

**5.** To return to sitting, roll to one side and slowly press up.

---

**Tip:** *This pose releases the low back and can stretch the backs of the legs and inner thighs for some people. If you cannot easily reach your big toes, hold on to your ankles instead, as in figure 2.10.*

# *Body Scan*
# AND TENSION RELEASE

**Total time: 5 minutes**

We will start each evening practice with this short awareness meditation, which will help you transition into your practice after the events of your day, release habitual tension, and prepare you for breathing. I encourage you not to skip this step. The internal integration that happens here is important to the success of the breathing practices that follow.

If you are new to sitting practices, your body scan will naturally last about three minutes, and you will then organically move on to the tension release. However, we are all different. You may find your timer alerts you before you have finished your scan, in which case you may need to extend your time, or you may adapt your scan to fit into the suggested period. As you become adept at this practice, you will no longer need your timer. With experience, you may wish to allow more time. To assist you in the beginning, you can listen to a guided audio recording at https://library.lumayoga.com/breathwork-body-scan.

The meditation has three parts:

**Awareness of the senses:** Use this time to reacquaint yourself with the sensory details you naturally filter out during your day. Guide your awareness sequentially from sense to sense, perhaps starting with sight, observing light and color even if the eyes are closed. Then move on to sound, taste, smell, and touch.

**Internal sensation:** The *inside* of your body contains a wealth of information in the form of sensations. I call this your "internal universe." These sensations, whether pleasurable, neutral, or unpleasant, constantly change. They can include aches and pains, awareness of hunger or satiation, physical sensations associated with emotion, and sensory feedback from our organs.

**Tension release:** Each day we gather and carry tension in our bodies. The third part of our meditation asks you to notice and consciously release tension where you hold it. Before you can move on to breathing, you must tune in to your body and notice and release residual tension.

## Part 1: Senses

**1.** Set your timer for 5 minutes.

**2.** Choose a comfortable position in which to sit, either in a chair or on the floor. You are also welcome to lie down, but be careful . . . you might fall asleep!

**3.** Start by becoming aware of your surroundings. If your eyes are open, take in the colors and shapes around you. If your eyes are closed, sense the light behind your eyelids. Become aware of the sounds in the room and the air against your skin. Observe the taste in your mouth. Take a few easy, long breaths and observe any smells in the room.

**4.** You have just tuned in to your *senses*. You are awake to where you are in time and space and to what's going on around you.

# Part 2: Internal Sensation

**1.** Next, turn your awareness in, toward your physical body. Find the bones and muscles of the hips, legs, and feet. Allow them to rest, heavy and supported. Notice the bones and muscles of the shoulders, arms, and hands. Allow your hands to relax. Completely relax your face. Relax the muscles of your jaw.

**2.** Begin to scan the body for other sensations. Where is there warmth? Where are you cool? Can you feel your circulation somewhere? Perhaps you can feel your pulse here or there or the beating of your heart. Sometimes we feel vibration, like a hum in the body. Some people "see" light or colors. Often, we become aware of aches and pains. Be sure also to notice the areas of the body where you are pain free. (There is always at least one place!)

**3.** Now you are awake to the kaleidoscope of sensations *inside* the body. Interoception is a special skill. It provides you with information about your *internal relationship* to where you are in time and space and to what's going on around you.

# Part 3: Tension Release

**1.** Without force, gently allow your breaths to become fuller. Encourage them to be smooth from the beginning of the breath to the end of the breath.

**2.** Bring your awareness to any tension you are holding. Pay special attention to tension in the shoulders, hands, and belly. Check for tension in your face and jaw. When you find tension, imagine it dissolving or melting away.

**3.** Maintaining a tall spine, continue to observe and resolve tension until you hear your timer alert you. If your eyes are closed, slowly open them and reorient yourself to the room. Observe how you feel.

---

**Tip:** *It's not uncommon to discover that we are agitated or anxious, especially those of us who tend to power through our days. With practice, we learn to see our agitation or anxiety simply for the emotions they are. Eventually we become able to release them. Alternately, you may find yourself feeling calm and relaxed. Regardless of your experience, if you have succeeded in noticing how you feel, you've succeeded in the work of the body scan.*

# The Eight Types of Breathing

I provided a brief description of the eight types of breathing in chapter 1. For more detailed information about breathing and breath types in general, I invite you to explore the resources listed in the last chapter, Conclusion: A Tool for Everyone (page 187). Briefly, however, let's review the eight types of breathing and learn more about why and how to integrate them into practice.

## Breath Awareness

The act of breathing is rich in sensory information that for the most part we take for granted. Breath awareness meditations invite us to slow down and enjoy the subtleties and nuances of our breathing. When we are successful, unrelated thoughts and preoccupations fade into the background, and we become completely engaged in the here and now—a goal of meditation.

The mind is like the Little Engine That Could. It just keeps going and going. One of the challenges of accessing a restful state of meditation is that it can be difficult to step off of the treadmill that is your thinking mind. Breath awareness gives the mind something to focus on. Inevitably your mind will wander, and you will have to repeatedly call it back to the task at hand. With practice, however, your mental focus will improve. As you become familiar with the way your mind works—its idiosyncrasies and rhythms—you will begin to differentiate the content of your thoughts from the part of you who is aware. Most people find this new perspective freeing. It releases us from the tension of constantly feeling the need to shape the reality before us and moves us toward appreciating our reality just as it is. What is unique about the breath, as opposed to other ways of engaging the mind, is that the breath is available to us as a point of focus in every moment.

If you're new to Breathwork, the simple act of paying attention to your breathing can sometimes make you feel as though you can't get enough air. If that happens for you, relax and notice that oxygen is abundant around you. It's everywhere!

## Belly Breaths

Belly breathing calms us, promoting PNS activation. If you struggle with anxiety, consider adding belly breathing into your day on a regular basis. In the midst of a panic attack, use it to help you regulate your nervous system. If you are angry, belly breathing can help you recover your center and resist the urge to shout something you might regret later. I start every breathing practice with a few belly breaths, regardless of my goals for the session.

Many have inherited a cultural ideal for what our bellies should look like. Whether for aesthetic purposes or due to stress, some people chronically tense their abdominal muscles. As you reconnect to this area of your body, consider that though we need to engage our abdominal muscles to support our movements, posture, and even breathing, there are times when we can let our abdominal muscles rest. Releasing chronic abdominal tension is integral to treating anxiety. It's not that the abdominals should always be relaxed when we breathe or that firming the abdominals is unhealthy. Our abdominals need to be free to engage and disengage as we need them, in support of the varied activities of our lives.

## Rib Cage Breathing

Rib cage breathing stimulates circulation and revitalizes the body, lifting our energy and our spirits. During rib cage breathing we employ the full capacity of the lungs. Normally, other than when we yawn, full use of the lungs is restricted to periods of intense exercise, acute SNS activation, or during the expression of intense emotion, such as when we laugh or sob. The rib cage also comes into motion when we experience intense pleasure, such as during orgasm.

If we make a habit of restricting rib cage movement for whatever reason, we may be limiting our potential to feel emotionally engaged. Enhancing our capacity for rib cage breathing is an act of enhancing our capacity to embrace life fully.

Learning the difference between belly breathing and rib cage breathing is foundational to being able to experience the nuance of Breathwork. They can be done in combination, as in the Breath Wave (page 59), or as an isolated practice, as in Horizon Breath (page 90). We will work with both variations.

## Resistance Breathing

As mentioned in chapter 1, traditional yoga breathing techniques use several methods for shaping the mouth and throat in order to create resistance to the air entering and leaving the lungs.

Vocalizations, such as singing or chanting, are by far the easiest and most accessible ways to engage with resistance breathing. When we are under stress, the throat often becomes restricted. Using sound to vibrate these tissues can help us let go of this tension. Singing and chanting in groups has been shown to cause a release of oxytocin, a hormone associated with happiness, bliss, and emotional bonding.

In Breathwork, resistance breathing is achieved by using the glottis as an aperture to narrow the throat passage as the air passes through, just as you do when you are whispering. In this way resistance can be applied to the in breath as well as the out breath. Teachers often describe the sound made by this style of breathing as similar to the sound of the ocean at the seashore or the wind in the trees. The sound we make by passing air with resistance through the throat is reminiscent of the sound we make when calming a baby—a correlation perhaps to the calming effect this breath has on the nervous system.

As you practice, you will notice that your breaths will naturally become slower and fuller. Be mindful to practice without hardness in the throat, and resist the tendency to clench your teeth or tense your jaw.

## The Breath Wave and Circular Breathing

The breath wave is the natural though subtle sequential movement of the spine that occurs when we breathe. Tuning in to this movement reveals the cyclical nature of breathing.

In Sanskrit, circular breathing is called *anulom valom*, which translates to "with the grain." The idea is that this breathing practice flows with, rather than contradicts, the natural expression of breathing in the body, therefore supporting the natural expression of our life force (prana) within us. Once a student is adept at *anulom valom*, adaptations can be made to the breath toward specific ends, such as balancing an internal disturbance or raising consciousness.

The circular breath moves *through* the steadiness of our seated posture like a great circular wave. The practice requires a conscious sequential coordination of all the organs, muscles, and systems physically responsible for breathing and uses all available lung space, from the lowest lobes up to the highest. When we breathe this way, we become entrenched in the cyclical nature of the breath cycle. Our breathing becomes less like a seesaw and more like the turning of a great Ferris wheel.

If any part of the breath wave is interrupted, it is an indication that we are bracing some part of the body and resisting the breath's natural flow. There is a time and place for bracing, such as when amplifying power, as during the Valsalva maneuver mentioned in chapter 1, or when applying certain breathing techniques, such as firming the belly during rib cage breathing. Chronic bracing, however, whether due to tension or emotional burden or for any other reason, even when subtle, is telling of a pattern we may wish to correct.

## Fast Breathing

Practitioners who are adept at fast breathing exercises can practice for several minutes without getting lightheaded or losing consciousness. The breath of fire, the fast breathing technique we use in Breathwork, is called *kapalabhati* in Sanskrit. This translates to "skull shining" and refers to the overall bright, vibrant, sometimes sparkly aspect that this breath elicits in us. After fast breathing, the body naturally wants to recover the appropriate saturation of $CO_2$ in the blood. The long, slow breaths of PNS activation come easily after such exercises.

As discussed, fast breathing can stimulate the SNS, which, in the absence of fear, can be energizing. In combination with other practices, fast breathing can be a beneficial component of a breathing regime, especially for people suffering from chronic fatigue or depression.

Start slowly. Later, you can increase both the pace and number of breaths you take. If ever you start to feel dizzy, tingly, numb, or faint during fast breathing, stop the practice and rest. Recover with full, slow breathing. The sensation should quickly pass.

## Alternate Nostril Breathing

Alternate nostril breathing is centering and helps us cultivate a sense of equanimity. Neuroscience links the right and left nostrils to left and right brain hemisphere activity respectively. The left hemisphere of the brain, associated with the SNS, is responsible for intellectual insight and logical problem solving, while the right is associated with the PNS and is responsible for intuition and creativity.

This breathing technique is very versatile. It can promote clarity, which can be beneficial for daytime activities, yet is easeful enough to practice in the evening before bed. Often one nostril is more congested than the other, usually due to the alternate swelling of erectile tissue in the turbinates. Those with a deviated septum can experience a disturbance to this rhythm that chronically prioritizes one nostril. We should not discount the ability of the human body to adapt, but the implications of nostril dominance might be something to consider when deciding whether to surgically correct a deviated septum.

## Timing and Suspending the Breath

Timings serve two purposes. First, similar to playing an instrument, they give the mind something rhythmic and mesmerizing to do. Second, as with music, the rhythmic and hypnotic patterns affect us in certain ways. Longer exhales are inherently settling. Even rhythms engender clarity and stability. Varied or uneven timings have an unnatural quality to them that causes us to become alert and pay attention.

We have already discussed the physical and emotional shifts that occur internally as a result of different kinds of breathing, but the very act of practicing provides a structure—a focus and a challenge—through which we might slip into a state of absorption. I once asked my yoga teacher in India about sitting for meditation. He said, "Do not sit for meditation. Sit for pranayama, and meditation will come naturally out of that."

Suspensions challenge us to become even more attentive during breathing. Have you ever noticed how a ball tossed into the air seems to hover for a moment, as if time is suspended, before gravity takes over and it begins its descent? If you can stay relaxed, suspending the breath can feel like that—an easeful pause, a moment of profound stillness in a noisy, busy world.

Through the lens of yoga, suspensions serve to arrest the natural flow of prana. During the disturbance, energetic conventions are dislodged, leaving, in theory, an internal environment conducive to the spontaneous awakening of latent life-force energy.

More practically, suspending the breath is an act of trust. In these moments we become confronted with the value of our breath and how precious it is to the continuation of life. To that end, if you try to hold your breath for longer than you're comfortable, suspensions will quickly become a source of suffering. Start where you are. If a suggested suspension feels too long, cut it in half. For example, if the technique asks you to hold for four counts, try holding for two. If that still feels too long, cut it in half again. Reduce your pause until suspending the breath feels easy, even if you've opted for a pause that lasts only for a heartbeat. *(If you are experiencing a more acute state of anxiety or you are in the midst of a panic attack, opt out of suspensions altogether.)*

Work to allow the pauses between breaths to be more like that suspended moment before the ball begins its descent and less like the gulp of air we take before going underwater. Each breath cycle has an arc. In essence, with suspensions, we are exploring comfortably lengthening the arc.

## Time to Begin

You now have everything you need to get started with Breathwork. Refer to this chapter any time you have questions or feel as though you'd like a little more information about the techniques in the exercises as I present them. Let's begin!

# PART TWO

## The Exercises

# Cultivating Integration

Now we begin our journey toward better breathing. This week, we'll focus on improving our physical selves through the breath. Besides helping us untangle our physical responses to stress, breathing techniques help us recapture our sense of *embodiment*. Conscious breathing reawakens us to the subtle rhythms and movements toward which our bodies naturally gravitate. Every moment we are breathing, the body is in motion. Stifle breath and you stifle movement. If you're less familiar with this concept, think about what you do with your body when you yawn or laugh. In this practice we work to reclaim our full capacity for breathing, which means we need to develop our capacity for full-body awareness.

As you move through this week, you may find yourself feeling better. You may even find you sleep better at night. Undoubtedly, you will also experience resistance. This is normal. Remind yourself that it's not always easy to engage with something new.

## Day 1

Integration happens when differentiated parts, each with their own purpose, work optimally together. Our first practices focus on developing breath awareness and remembering the different ways that we breathe.

*Morning Exercise:*
# RECLINED BELLY BREATHING

**Total time: 10 minutes**

Each morning, we will take the first few minutes of practice to prepare our bodies for breathing with the Breath Prep Stretch and Reset Sequence (page 43). After, our practice will either help us develop a specific skill or culminate in a technique we will take forward into future weeks.

**1.** Begin with the Breath Prep Stretch and Reset Sequence (page 43). This practice commonly takes 3 to 5 minutes.

**2.** Now, set your timer for 3 minutes. Lie on your back with the soles of your feet on the floor and your knees up. Rest the palms of your hands on your belly, as in figure 3.1.

**3.** Take a moment to consciously release tension in your body. Relax your shoulders. Relax the muscles of your face. Allow for several normal breath cycles, observing the natural characteristics of your breathing in this position.

**4.** Begin belly breathing: As you inhale, encourage the belly to rise into the palms of your hands. As you exhale, allow the belly to soften and fall. Imagine you have a balloon inside your belly, one that fills with air as you breathe in and empties as you breathe out.

**5.** Staying as relaxed as possible, continue until your timer alerts you that 3 minutes have passed.

**6.** To come out of the pose, slowly draw your knees into your chest, roll to one side, and return to a comfortable seated position.

**7.** Take a moment to reorient yourself. Notice how you feel.

**8.** Open your journal and record your practice.

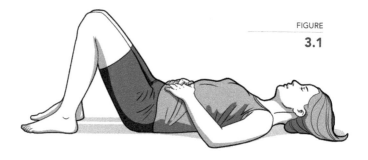

FIGURE

**3.1**

**Tip:** *The reclined position is good for getting started. In this position, belly breathing comes naturally. As you lie in preparation for today's practice, celebrate the soft nature of the belly when it is at rest. Observe how the belly naturally rises and falls as you breathe. As you experiment, recall what you learned about the diaphragm in chapter 1. With each inhale your abdominal organs are displaced by the phase 1 movement of the dia-phragm, causing your belly to rise. As the diaphragm relaxes, the organs return to their resting position.*

*Evening Exercise:*
# THE PATH OF THE BREATH

**Total time: 15 minutes**

Whereas our morning practices are devoted to promoting clarity, focus, and energy, our evening practices focus on integration and introspection. Each evening we will start with 3 to 5 minutes of the Body Scan and Tension Release meditation (page 52). Tonight, we follow with a visualization. To assist you in the beginning, you can listen to an audio recording at https://library.lumayoga.com/breathwork-path-of-the-breath.

## Steps

**1.** If possible, find a quiet place to practice and dim the lights. Find a comfortable position in which to sit. Refer to page 36 for tips on sitting comfortably for breathing.

**2.** Practice the Body Scan and Tension Release meditation. This practice commonly takes 3 to 5 minutes. If you are not using the online recording referenced in chapter 2 (page 52) for this meditation, set your timer for 5 minutes.

**3.** When the timer alerts you, stretch your legs, adjust your position, and return to your seated posture. Set your timer for another 5 minutes.

**4.** Shift your awareness to your breathing. Watch a few breaths come and go. Relax your shoulders, face, and jaw.

→

**5.** Follow the "path of your breath" through three phases:

» *Entry and exit*: Imagine that your nasal passages are caves. As you breathe in, visualize the air that enters the nose rolling in along the floor of the cave. As you breathe out, visualize the air that exits curling out along the roof of the cave. Notice that the breath is cooler as you draw it in and that it is warmer as it leaves the body. Follow this cycle for several breaths.

» *Inside the body*: As you inhale, follow the sweep of air through the throat and into the lungs. While you exhale, follow the breath back out again. Focus solely on the throat and lungs for several breaths.

» *Transitions*: Observe the moment your inhale turns to become an exhale and the moment your exhale turns to become an inhale. Focus solely on transitions for several breaths.

As you work through the phases, take your time. I recommend 7 to 10 breaths for each phase of the meditation.

**6.** With your remaining time, follow the complete path of the breath. Your breath appears to make a circle, traveling in one continuous loop: The breath travels in along the floor of the nostrils, through the throat, and into the lungs. The in breath transitions to an out breath, exits the lungs through the throat, and travels out along the roof of the nostrils. The out breath transitions to an in breath, then flows in again, etc.

**7.** When your timer alerts you that 5 minutes have passed, sit quietly for a moment. Notice how you feel.

**8.** Open your journal and record your practice.

---

**Tip:** *As your curiosity takes over during this meditation, you may notice that your breaths effortlessly become fuller and slower, so you have time to savor every moment of the experience. There is no right way to follow the path of the breath. However, I have suggested three areas to explore (entry and exit, inside the body, and transitions). Note how engaged the mind must become to follow the path of the breath. Note how easily the mind can become distracted.*

## Your Weekly Log: The Physical Body

Your journal is an excellent place to keep track of your progress. You won't know how you're progressing if you don't take a moment to record where you are today.

Quickly jot down a list of any physical concerns you may have. Examples might include pain, allergies, lack of sleep, or poor digestion. We will create a new list in week 2 for mood-related experiences like depression and anxiety. However, if you have *physical symptoms* that you associate with mood-related problems, list them as the physical symptoms that they are, here in week 1. For example, a sense of fatigue or heaviness could be due to depression. Instead of listing "feeling depressed," list the symptom itself: "physical fatigue and heavy limbs."

Next, list any physical issues that are more difficult to assess based on how you feel physically. Examples might be high blood pressure, high cholesterol, and diabetes. Though our breathing practice may or may not directly address the diseases and discomforts that can plague us, they are part of the big picture we have of our physical health that may be causing us concern.

Finally, if you have goals for physical performance, such as a desire to improve breathing for strength, endurance, or focus, list those.

Next to each physical concern, note how severe you feel your symptoms are on a scale of 1 to 10, with 10 being the most troublesome or inconvenient. Next to each performance goal, rate where you believe yourself to currently be on a scale of 1 to 10, with 10 representing having achieved your goal. We will revisit this log in a few days to note any changes.

## Day 2

Today we begin with rib cage breathing, which is naturally stimulating and energizing. When we fully engage the rib cage with our breath, we greatly increase the capacity of our lungs to take in air. Tonight we revisit belly breathing.

*Morning Exercise:*

# SEATED RIB CAGE BREATHING WITH STRAP

**Total time: 10 minutes**

This is a wonderful technique I learned from one of my breathing teachers, Max Strom. For part of this exercise, you will need a strap or belt with a fully adjustable buckle.

## Steps

**1.** Begin with the Breath Prep Stretch and Reset Sequence (page 43). Practice this for 3 to 5 minutes.

**2.** Secure the strap around your rib cage. Make sure the strap is at the level of the bottom tip of your breastbone, around the area of your solar plexus, as in figure 3.2. Tighten the strap so it is snug but doesn't feel overly restrictive.

→

**3.** Find a comfortable place to sit. Refer to page 36 for tips on sitting comfortably for breathing. Set your timer for 3 minutes.

**4.** Rest your hands on your lap. Relax your shoulders. Relax your face. Completely relax your jaw. Become aware of your breathing.

**5.** Start with a few rounds of belly breathing. You may notice the strap tightens around the ribs some as you breathe in and loosens as you breathe out. That means you are already moving the ribs a little with your breathing.

**6.** Transition to rib cage breathing: Without gripping or hardening your belly, firm your belly in and hold it there *as you continue to breathe*. With your belly firmed in as you breathe out, the strap will loosen around your ribs. With your belly firmed in as you breathe in, the strap will tighten around your ribs.

**7.** Use the strap for feedback to mobilize *only* your rib cage with your breathing. If your abdominal muscles are moving very little and you are feeling the tension of the strap increase with each in breath and loosen with each out breath, you are successfully rib cage breathing.

**8.** When the timer alerts you that 3 minutes have passed, remove the strap and sit quietly. Allow your belly to relax. Observe how you feel. Alternately, you may wish to lie down on your back for a few minutes, taking the position shown in figure 2.2 (page 38).

**9.** After your rest, open your journal and record your practice.

FIGURE
**3.2**

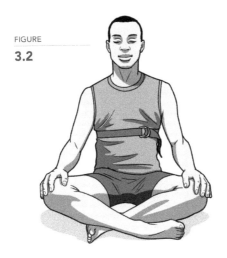

**Tip:** *So far as I know, Max is the only one who teaches rib cage breathing this way. I regularly offer it to my students, as I have found it to be an excellent teaching tool. Sometimes after rib cage breathing we can feel emotional. Max reminds his students that it is not the breathing practice that causes us to feel emotional; rather, deep breathing unearths stored emotions that we have yet to release and resolve. This is part of the healing process.*

*Evening Exercise:*

# PRONE BELLY BREATHING

**Total time: 10 minutes**

This excercise reminds me of the spontaneous and carefree rests children take between bouts of playing and running around. You may have naturally come into this breath while lying on your belly in the sun after a swim.

## Steps

**1.** Begin your evening practice with the Body Scan and Tension Release meditation (page 52). Then set your timer for 5 minutes.

**2.** Lie down on your belly. Fold your arms and rest your forehead on your forearms. Alternately, you may choose to lie with your arms alongside your body and your head turned to one side. Notice whether you generally favor turning your head in one direction. It is probably prudent to alternate sides each time you practice this breath.

**3.** Relax your body and bring your awareness to your breathing.

**4.** As you inhale, allow your belly to press down into the floor. As you exhale, let the belly soften. Like you did during Reclined Belly Breathing (page 68), take several breaths into the belly, as if the belly were a balloon you could fill with air.

**5.** As you breathe, observe the movement of your low back. With the in breath, the belly presses into the floor in order to expand, and your low back rises. As you breathe out, the low back falls.

**6.** As you breathe, observe the subtle rocking of your pelvis. With the in breath, the natural curve of the low back lessens. Consequently, the pelvis tilts slightly and the tailbone moves closer to the floor. When you exhale, the curve of the low back returns to its resting position, and the pelvis follows.

**7.** Take 10 to 12 more breaths here. Continue to notice the rise and fall of your low back and the gentle rocking of your pelvis. You do not need to encourage these movements. Let your breathing do the work. Your body is in motion *because* you are breathing.

**8.** When you have finished, center the head and neck, and slowly return to a comfortable seated position. Take a moment to notice how you feel.

**9.** Open your journal and record your practice.

---

**Tip:** *You probably have a very visceral familiarity with the comforting nature of these movements during your most relaxed and carefree moments, such as when you are dozing off to sleep or enjoying an excellent book.*

## Day 3

In order to work with breathing practices, we need to be able to better control how quickly or slowly the breath enters the body. Resistance breathing is a foundational tool for regulating the flow of breath. You will bring this technique into many of our future practices, including this evening's seated belly breathing.

*Morning Exercise:*
# RESISTANCE BREATHING

**Total time: 10 minutes**

Using resistance at the throat to slow the breath is as easy as fogging a mirror. You already do this every time you sigh or whisper. To assist you in the beginning, you can listen to an audio recording at http://library.lumayoga.com/breathwork-resistance-breathing.

**1.** Set your timer for 5 minutes and observe your breathing as you move through the Breath Prep Stretch and Reset Sequence (page 43).

**2.** Come to a comfortable seated position. Relax your shoulders. Relax your face, and relax your jaw.

**3.** Open your mouth and breathe out, as if you were going to fog your glasses in order to clean them. Take a breath in and repeat. Listen to the sound the breath makes as it passes along the throat. Pay attention to how the breath feels as it passes along the throat. Observe how you shape the glottis in order to make the *hhhhhhhh* sound.

**4.** Next, practice making the same sound with your in breath. This is less intuitive but requires the same shaping of the throat. Breathing through your mouth, work to make the sound of the in breath exactly the same as the sound you make when breathing out.

**5.** Set your timer for 3 minutes. With the mouth open, shape the throat in order to make a clear, even *hhhhhhhh* sound during both the in breath and the out breath.

**6.** Continue with resistance breathing until the timer alerts you that 3 minutes have passed. Return to normal breathing and sit quietly for another minute or two. Notice how you feel.

**7.** Open your journal and record your practice.

---

**Tip:** *Unlike a sigh, which starts heavy and fast and then trails off, work to make the sound of your breathing even and clear, as if you are singing a long* hhhhhhhh.

*Evening Exercise:*

# SEATED BELLY BREATHING

**Total time: 10 minutes**

Seated belly breathing is settling and supports the release of tension in
the belly, common to stress-related holding patterns.

## Steps

**1.** Set your timer for 5 minutes and begin the Body Scan and Tension
Release meditation (page 52). Observe and release tension wherever
you find it.

**2.** When your timer alerts you that 5 minutes have passed, stretch
your legs, adjust your position, and take a few deep breaths. Consider
holding one of those deep breaths in for a moment and then letting it
out with a great sigh.

**3.** Return to your seated position, and set your timer for 3 minutes.
Press down through the base of your pelvis in order to lift your spine
a little taller. At the same time, allow your shoulders to fall down and
away from your ears. Completely relax your hands and your face.

**4.** Exhale first and draw your belly in toward your spine. As you
breathe in, gradually relax your belly, letting it expand. As you breathe
out, as smoothly as you can, engage your abdominal muscles to draw
your belly back toward your spine.

**5.** Continue working with belly breathing. In the beginning it is difficult for the belly to move smoothly with your breath, and the process will feel uncoordinated. This is where resistance breathing can help.

**6.** Open your mouth and use resistance breathing in combination with belly breathing. Make the *hhhhhhhh* sound during both your inhale and your exhale. As you make the sound smooth, the movement of the belly will become smooth.

**7.** If at any point you start to feel agitated or frustrated *before* your timer rings, simply stop, rest, and start again. It takes time to build a sustained practice.

**8.** Continue until the timer alerts you that 3 minutes have passed. Return to normal breathing and sit quietly for a moment. Notice how you feel.

**9.** Open your journal and record your practice.

---

**Tip:** *Seated belly breathing takes some practice. Don't get discouraged if it's difficult to move the abdominals smoothly in and out.*

## Day 4

Today we pass the midpoint of the week, which presents an opportunity to take a broader view of how the breathing exercises are treating us. Consider taking an extra few minutes with your journal today to review your week so far.

*Morning Exercise:*
# RECLINED RIB CAGE BREATHING

**Total time: 10 minutes**

In this exercise, sensory feedback from the palms of your hands and from your ribs against the floor provides valuable information about how you are breathing.

## Steps

**1.** Begin with the Breath Prep Stretch and Reset Sequence (page 43). Practice this for 3 to 5 minutes.

**2.** Once your body scan is complete, lie down on your back with the soles of your feet on the floor and your knees up (figure 3.1, page 70.). Set your timer for 5 minutes.

**3.** Place your palms on your belly and take 5 Belly Breaths (page 57). Rest.

**4.** Shift your hands up to your low ribs. Slide the palms of your hands toward the sides of the rib cage, so your fingers are resting on your front bottom ribs and the heels of your hands are on either side of your rib cage, as in figure 3.3.

**5.** Begin rib cage breathing. Each time you breathe in, encourage your rib cage to broaden into the palms of your hands. Each time you breathe out, allow the rib cage to narrow. Take several breaths this way.

**6.** Keep your hands where they are, but shift your awareness to your back ribs. Each time you breathe in, encourage the back ribs to press down into the floor as they broaden. Each time you breathe out, observe the back ribs softening against the floor as they narrow.

**7.** Continue exploring rib cage breathing until the timer alerts you that 5 minutes have passed.

→

**8.** To come out of this position, slowly draw your knees into your chest, roll to one side, and return to a comfortable seated position. Breathe normally. Notice how you feel.

**9.** Open your journal and record your practice.

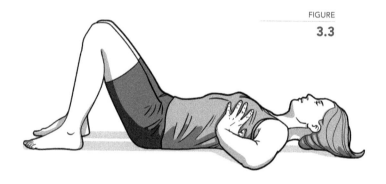

FIGURE

**3.3**

---

**Tip:** *Resting the hands on the ribs this way allows you to observe the movement of the front and sides of your rib cage at the same time. Make sure your palms are resting on the bones of the ribs, not the soft part of your belly or the sides of your waist. Work to actively move your rib cage when you breathe. Do your best to keep the belly as still as possible. Though it is not necessary for this exercise, you may find yourself spontaneously engaging with resistance breathing. Great!*

*Evening Exercise:*

# INTRO TO THE BREATH WAVE

**Total time: 15 to 20 minutes**

In this evening's practice we explore the sequential way in which our bodies naturally engage when we take full, deep breaths. You might want to come back to this practice a few times before moving on. We finish this practice with a short rest, allowing the body, mind, and nervous system time to integrate your work.

## Steps

**1.** Set your timer for 5 minutes and begin the Body Scan and Tension Release meditation (page 52). Observe and release tension in your body wherever you find it.

**2.** When the timer alerts you that 5 minutes have passed, lie down on your back with the soles of your feet on the floor and your knees up (figure 3.1, page 70). For the next few steps, you will count your breaths.

**3.** Place your palms on your belly and prepare to take 6 Belly Breaths (page 57). It can sometimes feel arresting to isolate your breathing to the belly alone. Stay as relaxed and as inquisitive as you can. Rest.

**4.** Shift your hands up to your low ribs. Slide the palms of the hands toward the sides of the rib cage, as you did during your morning practice (figure 3.3, page 86). Make sure your palms are resting on your bones, not the soft part of the belly or the sides of your waist.

**5.** Starting with a belly breath, continue to breathe in until the lower part of your rib cage under your palms starts to rise and broaden. When you are ready to exhale, exhale naturally; observe the rib cage returning to its starting position and your belly softening and releasing down toward the floor. Repeat for 5 more breaths. Rest.

**6.** Place your hands on your ribs as before. This time, you will fill the lungs further. Start your in breath by expanding your belly as instructed for belly breathing. As you draw more breath in, observe first your lower and then your middle rib cage expanding and broadening. As you exhale, observe the narrowing and relaxing of your rib cage and the softening and releasing of your abdominal muscles. Repeat for 5 more breaths. Rest.

**7.** Place your hands on your ribs as before. This time you will fill the lungs to capacity. Start your in breath by expanding your belly, as instructed for belly breathing. As you draw more breath in, observe first your lower and then your middle rib cage expanding and broadening. As you fill your lungs even further, your breastbone and collarbones will start to rise. When your lungs are full, pause for a moment, then begin your exhale. While you are exhaling, observe the fall of your collarbones and breastbone, the narrowing and relaxing of your rib cage, and the softening and releasing of your abdominal muscles.

**8.** Release your hands from your ribs and rest. Breathe normally.

**9.** Set your timer for 5 to 7 minutes and stretch out your legs. Consider sliding a rolled blanket or bolster under your thighs. If you are chilly, cover up with a blanket. Close your eyes. Scan your body for tension and release it when you find it. Settle in and enjoy.

**10.** When your timer alerts you, bring your knees in toward your chest and roll to one side. Slowly sit up and reorient yourself to the room. Notice how you feel.

**11.** Open your journal and record your practice.

---

**Tip:** *This exercise introduces us to the sequential nature of the bodily movements that are essential to deep, full breathing. I call this the "breath wave." As you practice, remind yourself to stay relaxed. Keep in mind that as you work toward engaging with your fullest possible breath, you can do so in a way that reinforces tension or reinforces ease.*

## Day 5

This morning we begin to apply the breathing vocabulary we have been developing to a technique that we will take forward into the coming weeks. Tonight we continue our play with the breath wave.

*Morning Exercise:*
# HORIZON BREATH

**Total time: 10 minutes**

Horizon breathing cultivates both stability and grace and connects us directly to a sense of energetic vitality. To assist you in the beginning, you can view a video tutorial at https://library.lumayoga.com /breathwork-horizon-breathing.

**1.** Set your timer for 5 minutes. This morning, challenge yourself to take full rib cage breaths as you move through the Breath Prep Stretch and Reset Sequence (page 43). Once you've finished, come to standing.

**2.** Secure your strap around your rib cage. Set your timer for 3 minutes.

**3.** Stand with your feet slightly wider than hip distance apart. Turn your feet so they are parallel and your toes are pointing forward. Bend your knees. Place your palms together in front of your chest. This is the starting position for the horizon breath—see figure 3.4.

FIGURE
**3.4**

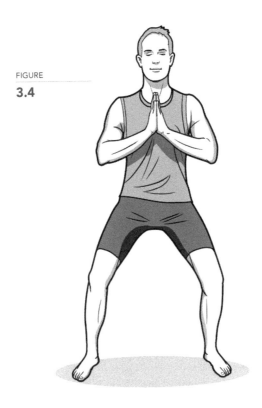

**4.** Exhale and firm your belly in.

**5.** Using rib cage breathing and resistance breathing, with your mouth open, inhale and open the arms out to the sides with the palms facing up (keep the elbows slightly bent and the shoulders down, as in figure 3.5).

→

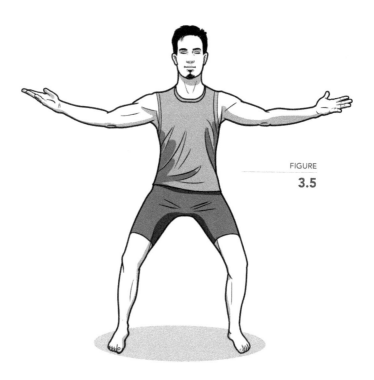

FIGURE
**3.5**

**6.** As you exhale, return to the starting position: Bring your palms back together in front of your breastbone.

**7.** Repeat steps 5 and 6 until the timer alerts you that 3 minutes have passed. Sit or lie down for a few minutes and observe the effects of your practice.

**8.** Open your journal and record your practice.

---

**Tip:** *As you coordinate your movement with your breathing, move slowly and evenly. Remember, the horizon breath is a rib cage breath (see page 18). Whereas the breath wave incorporates the coordination of all our breathing muscles, the rib cage breath restricts the diaphragm from dropping down and isolates breathing in the rib cage alone. In order to do this, you will need to firm your abdominal muscles in and keep them in while you are breathing. During rib cage breathing, the belly stays lifted and engaged.*

# Breath and Embodiment: Cultivating Integration

Our ability to feel internal sensations such as muscle soreness and temperature is associated with an area of the cerebral cortex called the *insula*. Not only does this region of the brain allow us to feel inside the body (interoception), it is also responsible for our ability to feel emotion as well as our sense of self, or consciousness.

The insula is a bilateral structure. The left insula, folded deep within the cerebral cortex of the left hemisphere, receives information from the parasympathetic nervous system (PNS) and is associated with positive feelings such as trust. The right insula is located within the right hemisphere of the brain and receives information from the sympathetic nervous system (SNS). It is associated with negative feelings such as mistrust.

The physical act of slow, deep breathing stimulates the PNS, which in turn stimulates the left insula, promoting positive emotions. The PNS and the left insula work in opposition to the SNS and the right insula. When one is active, the other turns off. Our ability to feel safe, empathize with others, and connect with one another is deeply enhanced when the PNS and the left insula are active.

We experience everything around us directly through our bodies. What we fail to recognize is how our breathing can actually affect how we *perceive* what we experience through our bodies. Mind-body integration is an act of aligning the information coming in through the senses with the internal information we gather through interoception.

*Evening Exercise:*
# PRONE BREATH WAVE

**Total time: 10 minutes**

You already have experience with how your pelvis, organs, and ribs come into motion when you breathe. With this exercise, we spend a little more time with the spine.

## Steps

**1.** Set your timer for 5 minutes. Get comfortable in your sitting posture, and begin your Body Scan and Tension Release meditation (page 52). If you have extra time after your scan, focus your mind on your breathing and on the subtle body movements that occur as you breathe.

**2.** When you've finished your scan, set your timer for another 5 minutes. Lie down on your belly. Take 5 to 7 prone Belly Breaths (page 57). Observe the rise and fall of your low back. Observe the subtle rocking of your pelvis.

$\longrightarrow$

**3.** If your head is turned, change sides for 5 to 7 more breaths. This time, encourage your breathing to become longer and fuller. In order to take fuller breaths, your lower back ribs and then the middle part of the back of your rib cage, in that order, will naturally come into motion. Because the ribs are attached to the spine, the spine then also comes into motion. The reverse happens when you exhale.

**4.** Turn your head once again and take a few more breaths. This time *encourage* the breath to "wave" through the spine: As you breathe in, first the pelvis begins to tilt, then the low back rises, then the low ribs followed by the mid-ribs come into motion. If you continue to fill the lungs, the ribs toward the base of the neck will come into motion. If the lungs fill all the way, it might even feel natural to lift the head slightly and allow the breath wave to sequence through the cervical spine. As you exhale, observe the "wave" naturally reversing.

**5.** Continue exploring the breath wave. Make these last prone breaths as subtle or as deep as you would like them to be.

**6.** When the timer alerts you that 5 minutes have passed, slowly return to a comfortable seated position. Take a minute or two to reorient yourself to the room. Notice how you feel.

**7.** Open your journal and record your practice.

## Day 6

You now have direct experience with the three separate components of holistic breathing that make up the foundational practices of Breathwork: belly breathing, rib cage breathing, and the breath wave. This represents a solid base from which to move forward. Let's play!

*Morning Exercise:*
# HORIZON BREATH REFINED

**Total time: 10 minutes**

This morning we practice horizon breathing without the strap and further refine our approach.

## Steps

**1.** Set your timer for 5 minutes. Challenge yourself to use resistance breathing as you move through the Breath Prep Stretch and Reset Sequence (page 43). Take smooth, even breaths.

**2.** Come to standing and prepare for Horizon Breath (page 90). Set your timer for 3 minutes. Lift your belly in and up. Keep it in the entire time you are engaged in this breathing practice.

**3.** Begin horizon breathing. Remember to use both rib cage breathing and resistance breathing. Breathe through your mouth, making the *hhhhhhh* sound during both your inhale and your exhale.

→

**4.** Once you get comfortable with the rhythm, sound, and coordinated movements of the breath, imagine you are wearing the strap around your rib cage.

**5.** Each time you breathe in, focus on expanding the rib cage in all directions, just like you did when you were wearing the strap. Focus your breath into the side ribs and back ribs as well as the front chest.

**6.** When you breathe out, consciously narrow and condense the rib cage back toward center and your starting position.

**7.** Continue practicing horizon breathing until your timer alerts you that 3 minutes have passed. Step your feet together and stand quietly for a moment. Observe how you feel.

---

**Tip:** *Horizon breathing is a rib cage breath, which means it is stimulating. This is why we practice it in the morning. If at any time you feel dizzy or lightheaded during this exercise, bend your knees and fold forward from the hips. Putting your head down should immediately relieve the symptoms. To return to standing, look up first. Leading with the head, slowly return to vertical.*

*Evening Exercise:*

# OPENING THE CHEST + RECLINED BREATH WAVE

**Total time: 15 to 20 minutes**

Tonight we take a break from our usual body scan meditation in order to spend more time with this breathing practice. To assist you in the beginning, you can listen to an audio recording of reclined breath wave at https://library.lumayoga.com/breathwork-reclined-breath-wave.

## Steps

**1.** Fold your blanket in preparation for Opening the Chest Reclined Posture (page 40). Set your timer for 15 minutes and come into the posture.

**2.** As the posture stretches the front of the rib cage, you will notice your breathing is affected. Allow the belly to rise and fall naturally with the breath. Take 5 to 7 Belly Breaths (page 57), observing the subtle shift of the low back and pelvis as you breathe.

**3.** After 5 to 7 Belly Breaths, explore 5 to 7 slightly deeper breaths, encouraging the lower rib cage to become engaged with your breathing. When you breathe out, imagine your exhale sliding down the back surface of your body toward your toes.

→

**4.** Once you feel established in the breathing in the belly to the lower rib cage, take 5 to 7 slightly deeper breaths, encouraging the middle chest and side ribs to open to receive each in breath. When you breathe out, imagine your exhale sliding down the back surface of your body toward your toes.

**5.** Pause and check in. This might be plenty for now. If you feel at all anxious, agitated, or short of breath, skip to step 7; otherwise carry on with step 6.

**6.** Prepare for 2 to 3 more breath waves. This time, experiment with using all your lung capacity: With your inhale, allow the belly to rise, followed by the low ribs. As the lungs fill, the middle chest will rise, and the side ribs will broaden. Finally, as the lungs reach capacity, the upper chest and collarbones will come into motion. When you reach the top of the breath, pause for a heartbeat. As you breathe out, imagine your exhale sliding down the back surface of your body toward your toes.

**7.** When you've finished, rest quietly until your timer alerts you to end your practice.

**8.** Exit the posture slowly. Roll off your blanket to one side and rest here. As you feel ready, press up to a sitting position and orient yourself to the room. Notice how you feel.

**9.** Open your journal and record your practice.

---

**Tip:** *Opening the chest is a direct and powerful contradiction to the body's natural positional reaction to stress, which is to curl the shoulders forward and hunch over in a defensive posture. The movement of the in breath from belly to collarbones expands the thoracic cavity sequentially, engaging every muscle and organ responsible for breathing. As you work with deep breathing, staying relaxed is key. You may find yourself naturally using resistance breathing to help you better control both the ascent and the descent of the wave.*

*Pay special attention to how you feel after tonight's practice. This exercise can be stimulating, but the longer rest should help you transition effortlessly to sleep. Be gentle with yourself this evening. Emotional shifts tend to occur during or after deep breathing.*

# Document your progress!

You may remember, or you could look up your previous baseline to compare your progress. Keep in mind, however, that after only six days this is not yet a true gauge of your progress. You need more data. Reflect on your experience this week with integrating a regular breathing practice into your life. Look through the lens of your physical experience of breathing.

»   Overall, how has it been to work with your breath twice a day?

»   Has Breathwork helped you become more aware of your physical body this week?

»   Which exercises come easily? Which exercises are more challenging? Why?

»   Do you prefer the morning practice or the evening?

»   How have you been sleeping?

»   What are your fears?

»   What are your doubts?

»   Is there anything else that has been going on for you that might be worth writing down here?

## Day 7

Welcome to day 7! You are well on your way to establishing a regular breathing practice. Today we reassess our progress by returning to the 3-minute baseline exercise from chapter 1. Tonight we revisit the path of the breath awareness meditation in a resting posture that is deeply restorative for the low back.

*Morning Exercise:*
# 3-MINUTE BASELINE

**Total time: 10 to 12 minutes**

Use your new skills of breath awareness to tune in to each breath and stay with it from the beginning of the cycle to the end. If at all possible, *enjoy* this exercise!

## Steps

**1.** Set your timer for 5 minutes. Challenge yourself to take smooth, even resistance breaths as you move through the Breath Prep Stretch and Reset Sequence (page 43).

**2.** Come to a comfortable seated position and set your timer for 3 minutes.

**3.** Close your eyes and begin to count your breaths. Resist the urge to actively try to take fewer breaths. Your only job this morning is to take full, comfortable breaths at a comfortable and easily manageable pace.

## Steps (cont.)

**4.** When your timer alerts you that 3 minutes have passed, make a mental note of how many breaths you've taken. Return to normal breathing. Notice how you feel.

**5.** Pull out your journal and record the number of breaths you took in 3 minutes.

*Evening Exercise:*

# REST AND RESET +
# THE PATH OF THE BREATH

**Total time: 15 to 20 minutes**

Tonight we take a break from active breathing exercises and return to developing breath awareness. Get your journal handy. We'll start with journaling so that after our rest and reset practice, we can more easily remain in what should be a delicious, easeful, and relaxed state.

## Steps

**1.** Pull out your weekly log. Review your list of the physical concerns you recorded at the beginning of the week. Next to each item on the list, note how severe you feel your symptoms have been on a scale of 1 to 10 since your last assessment (10 being the most troublesome, severe, or inconvenient). Review your goals, keeping in mind that you are only 7 days into your breathing routine. Record any other observations, ideas, or insights worth noting as you wrap up week 1.

→

**2.** Set your timer for 10 minutes. Lie down on your back with your legs up the wall, as shown in figure 3.6. If your hamstrings are tight and your knees cannot straighten, simply move away from the wall and come into the variation shown in figure 3.7.

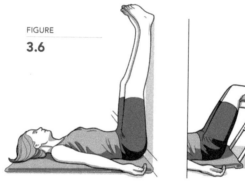
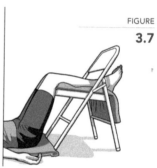

FIGURE
**3.6**

FIGURE
**3.7**

**3.** Allow your arms to rest away from your body. Move your shoulders down and away from your ears. Close your eyes.

**4.** Bring your awareness to your breath. Allow your breathing to occur naturally, and observe a few breaths as they come and go.

**5.** Gently shift your focus to the path of the breath (page 71). Follow your breath through its entry and exit at the nostrils, its journey inside and out of your body, and the transitions between breaths. Take your time.

**6.** After a minute or two, you may find your mind wandering. At first, call your mind back to the path of the breath. Gently encourage your mind to stay with the meditation. Each time you notice the mind wandering, like a fisherman reeling in a net, patiently reel the mind back to your breath.

**7.** After some time, if a dreamlike sleep state washes over you, accept it and allow your body to settle more and more deeply into relaxation. However, if your mind turns toward worrying, problem solving, or rehashing past events, continue to guide the mind back to your breathing.

**8.** When your timer alerts you that 10 minutes have passed, slowly draw your knees into your chest, roll to one side, and return to a comfortable seated position. Notice how you feel.

**9.** To finish your practice this evening, place a palm over your heart and appreciate the soft rise and fall of your chest as you breathe. Take a moment to cultivate a sense of gratitude for your breath and how it enlivens you every single day.

---

**Tip:** *Celebrate your heightened awareness of the different movements and sensations of breathing. Notice the sense of ease that follows some of the exercises. This is the feeling of having integrated, through conscious practice, breath, mind, and body. Breathing consciously is not only physically nourishing but can also be deeply soul satisfying. Breathing is nothing less than an act of communing with the pure, life-sustaining radiance that exists within each of us.*

# Cultivating Awareness

As our bodies disentangle from the holding patterns that help us cope with life's challenges and we learn to let go and allow for breathing, we become more sensitive to the relationship between our inner world and how we interact with the world around us. Inevitably, self-awareness surfaces, and opportunities for reflection arise. It is common to find ourselves in a different mental state from when we began or enjoying periods of enhanced mental clarity and calm. Sometimes our practice reveals and helps us integrate suppressed emotions and persistent worldviews that no longer serve us.

This week we will continue to refine the breathing tools introduced in week 1. We will now shift our focus, however, toward experiencing Breathwork through the lens of *mind* and *mood*.

## Day 1

As you work with repetition, you will start to feel more confident in the techniques of Breathwork. At the same time, you may start to favor one practice over another. For now, unless there is a reason not to (see page 34), stay with the program as presented. After week 3, you can tailor the practice to your preferences and needs.

*Morning Exercise:*

# HORIZON BREATH, BREATH INITIATED MOVEMENT

**Total time: 10 minutes**

Coordinating movement and breath increases mental focus and enhances muscular coordination. With this practice we reinvest in the deep, organic mind-body connection we started to experience in week 1.

*Steps*

**1.** Begin your morning practice with the Breath Prep Stretch and Reset Sequence (page 43).

**2.** Come to standing and prepare for Horizon Breath (page 90).

**3.** Set your timer for 3 minutes, and begin horizon breathing. Once you have established a comfortable rhythm, continue to step 4.

**4.** Shift your focus slightly. Rather than *coordinating* the movements of your arms with the movements of your rib cage and lungs, move as though your arms are *motivated* by your breathing.

**5.** When your timer alerts you that you have been breathing consciously for 3 minutes, step your feet together and stand quietly for a moment. Observe how you feel.

**6.** Open your journal and record your practice.

---

**Tip:** *This moving meditation is called* breath initiated movement, *and it takes some practice! Like tuning an instrument, breath initiated movement during horizon breathing brings the mind, body, and breath into synchronicity. As you refine this exercise, imagine the action of the arms is inspired by the action of the lungs. In this way, the breath will lead and the movement will follow ever so slightly behind. If breath initiated movement felt awkward today, keep practicing. Soon it will be second nature. To assist you in the beginning, you can view a video tutorial at https:// library.lumayoga.com/breathwork-breath-initiated-movement.*

*Evening Exercise:*

# THE BREATH WAVE, FULL CIRCLE

**Total time: 10 minutes**

Tonight we learn what is considered the foundation of yoga pranayama, often referred to as circular breathing.

## Steps

**1.** Set your timer for 5 minutes and come to a comfortable seated position for the Body Scan and Tension Release meditation (page 52). You have probably started to notice that there are specific areas where you store tension. Observe and release the tension in your body wherever you find it.

**2.** Stretch your legs and adjust your posture in preparation for another 3 minutes of seated practice. Set your timer and close your eyes.

**3.** Begin with a few grounding Belly Breaths (page 57): Round and expand your belly as you breathe in. Draw your belly back toward your spine as you breathe out. Take 5 breaths this way.

**4.** Continue with belly breathing, but gradually allow the breaths to become slightly fuller so the low ribs become mobile: Start with the movement of your belly as you begin your in breath. After the belly expands, continue breathing in and witness the low ribs expand. As you breathe out, empty the low ribs first and then draw your belly in. Take 5 breaths this way.

**5.** Begin as you did in step 4, but gradually allow the breaths to become even fuller so the mid-chest, side ribs, and back ribs become mobile: Start with the movement of the belly as you begin your in breath. As the lungs continue to fill, allow the low ribs to expand. As the lungs fill further, the mid-chest, side ribs, and mid-back ribs will expand. As you breathe out, empty in reverse order, starting with the mid-chest, side ribs, and back ribs. Follow with the low ribs. Toward the end of the out breath, draw the belly in. You are now fully engaged with the breath wave during your exhale as well as your inhale and have transitioned into circular breathing. Take 5 breaths this way.

**6.** Pause now to observe whether you are feeling agitated or tense. Relax your face. Let your shoulders fall down and away from your ears. Completely relax your hands. Even subtle frustration, agitation, or shortness of breath can be an indication that you have reached your capacity for today.

**7.** Return to belly breathing, and for the remainder of your time allow the grounding and centering nature of this breath to calm and stabilize you.

**8.** When your timer alerts you that 3 minutes have passed, return to normal breathing. Sit quietly for another minute or so. Observe how you feel.

**9.** Open your journal and record your practice.

---

**Tip:** *Posture is important here. Without rigidity, maintain a tall spine throughout. It might help to imagine that you are filling your torso with breath as you would fill a glass with water: from bottom to top. One or two full circular breaths might be enough in the beginning. Remember the importance of staying relaxed, and feel free to take breaks between breaths. Over time you will develop the ability to sit for longer and engage in a continuous practice of circular breathing.*

## Your Weekly Log: Mind and Mood

This week, list any mental or emotional concerns you have. Examples might include mental fatigue, spaciness, or forgetfulness or overall mood tones such as the blues, depression, or lack of motivation. Include any struggles with insomnia, social anxiety, or panic attacks as well as any unpleasant preoccupying thoughts, such as challenges you face at work, concerns about loved ones, or looming responsibilities. Not everyone has concerns such as these, but many of us do. List anything that occurs to you.

Separately, list any goals you have for improving mental functioning or mood. For example, you might have a specific goal to process grief from the loss of a loved one. Or perhaps you are a slow starter in the morning, and you hope to use breathing to feel more awake in the first hours of the day. Some people wish to shed a persistent fear of inadequacy or other harmful self-judgments.

Next to each concern, note how severe you feel it is on a scale of 1 to 10, with 10 being the most troublesome or inconvenient. Next to each goal, rate where you believe yourself to currently be on a scale of 1 to 10, with 10 representing having achieved your goal. We will revisit this log in a few days to note any changes.

## Day 2

Today we add two new breathing techniques to our toolbox: fast breathing, which lifts energy and with it our mood, and alternate nostril breathing, which helps us access opposing qualities within ourselves. We can use these breaths in different ways to recalibrate when we've been thrown off-center.

*Morning Practice:*

# BREATH OF FIRE

**Total time: 10 minutes**

Fast breathing temporarily alters $CO_2$ levels in the body. Slow, controlled breaths come more easily after fast breathing. To assist you in the beginning, you can view a video tutorial at https://library.lumayoga.com/breathwork-breath-of-fire.

**1.** Begin your practice with the Breath Prep Stretch and Reset Sequence (page 43). Practice with Rib Cage Breathing (page 18) and Resistance Breathing (page 58). Notice how this more dynamic breath, though long and full, is both warming and stimulating.

**2.** Come to a comfortable seated position in preparation for 3 rounds of the breath of fire. You do not need your timer for this exercise.

**3.** Recall Belly Breaths (page 57). Breath of fire is a belly breath. However, during this fast breathing technique the belly "snaps" quickly in toward the spine to force a rapid exhale. Exhales become short successive blasts or puffs of air. These breaths happen in rapid succession.

**4.** This is how to do it:

» Sit tall and relax your shoulders.

» Take about half a breath in. Let your belly round as in belly breathing.

» Rapidly and with force, pull your belly in toward your spine and exhale at the same time. The breath will leave the nostrils in a fast outward puff of air.

» Immediately after your exhale, relax the belly and let the inhale occur as a natural rebound to the out breath. In other words, focus on each exhale, and let your inhale happen all by itself. As the belly relaxes, your breath will come into the nostrils without effort.

» Continue in rapid succession at a pace somewhere between 1 and 2 breaths per second. Later you may increase this pace.

**5.** Start with 3 rounds of 12 breaths. As you become more comfortable, work up to 30 breaths per round. Between rounds, pause and breathe normally. We call these "recovery breaths."

→

**6.** When you have finished 3 rounds of the breath of fire, sit quietly for another minute or two. Observe how you feel.

**7.** Record your practice.

---

**Tip:** *During fast breathing we are essentially hyperventilating. This style of breathing can make you feel lightheaded when you're not used to it. A little lightheadedness is to be expected, but if you get dizzy or your hands start to tingle, stop immediately and take several normal breaths. The symptoms should resolve quickly.*

*Evening Exercise:*

# ALTERNATE NOSTRIL BREATHING

**Total time: 10 minutes**

This version of alternate nostril breathing supports balance and equanimity in both mind and mood. To assist you in the beginning, you can view a video tutorial at https://library.lumayoga.com /breathwork-alternate-nostril.

## Steps

**1.** Come to a comfortable seated position and set your timer for 5 minutes. Practice the Body Scan and Tension Release meditation (page 52).

**2.** When you have finished your scan, stretch your legs and adjust your position in preparation for 3 more minutes of seated breathing practice.

**3.** Set your timer. Close your eyes. Relax your shoulders. Relax your jaw. Completely relax your hands. Begin taking long, smooth breaths.

**4.** Hold up your right hand and fold your index and second fingers in toward your palm.

**5.** With the thumb of your right hand, close off your right nostril so no air can pass through. Exhale through your left nostril.

→

**6.** Take a long, smooth breath in through your left nostril.

**7.** When the lungs are full, use your ring finger to close off your left nostril, and exhale through your right nostril.

**8.** Take a long, smooth breath in through your right nostril. At the top of the breath, when the lungs are full, use your thumb to close off your right nostril and exhale through your left.

**9.** Continue, switching nostrils after each inhale.

**10.** If at any point in the practice you start to feel agitated, frustrated, or short of breath, simply stop to rest. Take a few recovery breaths. Then start again.

**11.** When your timer alerts you that 3 minutes have passed, continue with your current breath cycle until you finish an exhale through your left nostril.

**12.** Release your right hand to your lap and return to normal breathing. Sit quietly for another minute or two. Notice how you feel.

**13.** Record your practice.

---

**Tip:** *It is not unusual to experience a sense of emotional poise and/or physical grace after the practice of alternate nostril breathing. Sometimes we find that a solution to a problem we've been mulling over spontaneously reveals itself to us. We often spend much of our day leaning on the role of one brain hemisphere over the other. For example, as I sit to write this, my left brain is dominant, working to put concepts into language. Practicing alternate nostril breathing alternately stimulates opposite hemispheres, promoting communication between the two sides of the brain.*

## Day 3

Clear, even breaths help us feel vibrant, alive, and mentally focused. This morning we will work to hone and refine horizon breathing by using a *timing*. Tonight, we'll reinforce the natural wavelike nature of breathing by revisiting the circular breathing technique.

*Morning Exercise:*

# 4:4 HORIZON BREATH, HONING YOUR RHYTHM

**Total time: 10 minutes**

Assigning a count to the breath helps us adjust the pace and rhythm or "timing" of our breathing. To assist you in the beginning, you can listen to an audio recording of this exercise on https://library.lumayoga.com /breathwork-4-4-horizon-breathing.

## Steps

**1.** Begin your morning practice with the Breath Prep Stretch and Reset Sequence (page 43). Resist the urge to rush. Use this time to set the tone for your practice.

**2.** Come to standing, set your timer for 3 minutes, and prepare for Horizon Breath (page 90).

**3.** Steady your gaze. Softly focus your eyes on something in front of you, or close your eyes.

**4.** Begin horizon breathing. As you practice, add the following 4:4 timing to your breath: Count to 4 as you breathe in. Count to 4 as you breathe out. It's that simple.

**5.** When your timer alerts you that 3 minutes have passed, step your feet together and stand quietly for a moment. Observe how you feel. Consider sitting or lying down for a few minutes to rest.

**6.** Record your practice.

---

**Tip:** *To get the most out of this exercise, count at a comfortable, even pace (like the beating of a steady drum), take full breaths, and practice resistance breathing with the mouth open. Make the same sound during your inhale as you make during your exhale.*

*Evening Practice:*

# CIRCULAR BREATHING, HONING YOUR TECHNIQUE

**Total time: 15 to 20 minutes**

A practice is just that: *practice*. Keep it simple. Here, we revisit the Breath Wave, Full Circle from page 112. Tonight, experiment with using your full lung capacity.

*Steps*

**1.** Set your timer for 5 minutes and come to a comfortable seated position for the Body Scan and Tension Release meditation (page 52). Tune in to your senses. Tune in to your body. Actively let go of the tension you have collected during your day.

**2.** After your scan, stretch your legs and adjust your posture. Set your timer for another 5 minutes of seated breathing practice. Close your eyes. Start your breathing practice with a few grounding Belly Breaths (page 57).

**3.** Begin circular breathing by breathing into your belly, as if your belly were a balloon you could fill with air. Continue to breathe in until the low ribs expand with the breath. When it's time to breathe out, empty the low ribs first and then draw the belly in. Take 5 breaths like this.

**4.** Repeat step 3. This time, however, extend your in breath until the mid-chest, side ribs, and area around the heart expand with the breath. When it's time to breathe out, empty the mid-chest, side ribs, and area around the heart first, then the low ribs, and last, draw the belly in. Take 5 breaths like this.

**5.** Finally, so long as you are not feeling agitated, frustrated, or short of breath, continue working with circular breathing as described in step 4. This time, however, extend your in breath until the upper chest and area under the collarbones fill with breath and the lungs are full. When it's time to breathe out, empty the upper chest and area under the collarbones first, then the mid-chest and area around the heart, then the low ribs, and last, draw the belly in. Sometimes just 1 or 2 breaths like this is enough.

**6.** Pause now to observe whether you became agitated or tense during your breathing. Relax your face. Let your shoulders fall down and away from your ears.

**7.** For your remaining practice time, continue with circular breathing. If you are feeling most comfortable with the version in step 3 or step 4 rather than the full-breath version as described in step 5, stick with the version you're comfortable with for now.

**8.** When your timer alerts you that 5 minutes have passed, complete your current breath cycle, ending with your next exhale. Return to normal breathing and stay seated for another minute or two. Notice how you feel.

**9.** Set your timer, and lie down to rest for 5 to 10 minutes.

**10.** After your rest, draw your knees in toward you, roll to one side, and return to sitting. Record your practice.

---

**Tip:** *I strongly encourage you to allow yourself the short rest suggested in step 9 as part of your practice. Not only does this give you an opportunity to observe the effects of your efforts, it provides your nervous system valuable time to integrate any internal shift and recalibrate.*

## Day 4

As we continue to build on our Breathwork vocabulary, we will now begin to combine techniques so our morning and evening sessions come to resemble more complete breathing practices. With this morning's practice we pass the midpoint of week 2 and reach the halfway mark of our 21-day experience! Today I have included an optional bonus afternoon practice.

*Morning Exercise:*
# BREATH OF FIRE + VOCALIZATION

**Total time: 10 minutes**

Because many wish to avoid appropriating another culture's spiritual practice (such as chanting "om" in the yoga tradition), when practicing vocalizations we will simply use the vowel sounds *ah, a,* and *o.* To assist you in the beginning, you can view a video tutorial at https://library.lumayoga.com/breathwork-vocalization.

*Steps*

**1.** Begin your morning practice with the Breath Prep Stretch and Reset Sequence (page 43). Practice with both rib cage breathing and resistance breathing. ➞

**2.** Come to sitting for Breath of Fire (page 116). Complete 3 rounds of 12 to 30 breaths per round. (As your practice progresses, gradually work toward 3 rounds of 30 breaths.) Take recovery breaths between rounds, checking for and releasing any tension in your body and observing how you feel.

**3.** Stretch your legs and adjust your posture for a few more minutes of seated breathing. Set your timer for 3 minutes. Sit tall but relax your shoulders down and away from your ears, and let go of any tension in your hands and jaw. We will now slow down our breathing by using specific vocalizations.

**4.** Take a full breath in. Open your mouth and at a comfortable pitch for you (not too high but not too low), vocalize a long, steady *ahhhhhh* sound. The sound is the same as the *a* in *talk*. Keep vocalizing until you run out of breath.

**5.** Take another full breath and repeat *ahhhhhhhhh*. As you chant, notice where in the torso you most feel the vibration of the vocalization. Is the sound coming more from your belly, chest, or throat?

**6.** Next, continue vocalizing but change the sound to *a* as in *make*. Keep vocalizing until you run out of breath.

**7.** Repeat. Where do you feel the vibration now? It may have shifted to a different place in your body.

**8.** Finally, continue vocalizing but change the vowel sound to *o* as in *stone*.

**9.** Repeat. Where do you feel the vibration when you chant *o*?

**10.** Continue playing with vocalizations until your timer alerts you that 3 minutes have passed. Return to normal breathing and sit quietly for another minute or two. How do you feel?

**11.** Record your practice.

---

**Tip:** *Many people feel shy about using their voices. Vocalizing, as when we sing or chant, is the single easiest way to slow down the outgoing breath. Longer exhales calm us. If you are feeling hesitant about this exercise, do it in the service of experiencing your longest possible exhale. Vocalizations are simply resistance breathing in disguise.*

*Optional Afternoon Exercise:*

# LION'S BREATH

**Total time: 1 minute**

Consider this fun and fast cleansing breath when you need a quick shift in perspective or a pick-me-up when you find yourself lagging. To assist you in the beginning, you can view a video tutorial at https://library.lumayoga.com/breathwork-lions-breath.

## Steps

**1.** Come to a comfortable seated position. Close your eyes. Tune in to what is going on in your body right now, as you sit, in this moment. Tune in to what is going on in your mind. Tune in to anything that is present for you emotionally—not in general, just now in this moment.

**2.** Take a huge, full breath in. Fill the lungs all the way up to the top. When you think your lungs are full, pause for a moment, then try to take a little more breath in.

**3.** With great force, open your mouth and blast the air out of your lungs. As you do, open your eyes wide and stick out your tongue as far as it will go. Be loud. Be fierce. After all, this is called Lion's Breath.

**4.** Repeat twice more, for a total of 3 lion's breaths.

**5.** Close your eyes. Tune back in to your body, mind, and emotions. You might even find yourself smiling a little.

---

**Tip:** *If you spend your afternoons at a workplace, try to find some privacy, perhaps in a restroom or in your car. If you work in an office, you can sometimes find a few minutes for practice in an unused conference room. Be careful when practicing this breath around others; you will quickly clear the room!*

# REFINED ALTERNATE NOSTRIL BREATHING

**Total time: 15 to 20 minutes**

You may remember that circular breathing is considered the foundation of all yoga pranayama. Here, we refine alternate nostril breathing by adding circular breathing to the technique.

## Steps

**1.** We will start with seated practice and end with the Opening the Chest Reclined Posture (figure 2.5, page 42). Set up your folded blankets or bolster, so the support will be waiting for you when you're ready to lie down later.

**2.** Come to a comfortable seated position and set your timer for 5 minutes. Practice the Body Scan and Tension Release meditation (page 52).

**3.** When you have finished your scan, stretch your legs and adjust your position in preparation for 4 minutes of seated breathing practice.

**4.** Set your timer. Close your eyes. Relax your shoulders. Relax your jaw. Completely relax your hands. Take a few long, smooth breaths.

**5.** Begin Circular Breathing (page 124). Take 7 to 10 circular breaths.

**6.** Add Alternate Nostril Breathing to circular breathing. Begin with an exhale through the left nostril as described on page 19. Change nostrils after each inhale.

**7.** When your timer alerts you that 4 minutes have passed, continue through the cycle until you complete the next exhale through your left nostril.

**8.** Release your right hand to your lap and return to normal breathing. Sit quietly for another minute or two. Notice the physical sensations in your body. Notice your state of mind: Are you calm? Agitated? Alert? Sleepy?

→

**9.** Set your timer for another 5 to 10 minutes. Lie down on your support. Check to make sure your head is supported and your arms are away from your body. Rest.

**10.** When your timer alerts you to end your rest, exit the posture slowly by rolling to one side and returning to sitting.

**11.** Record your practice.

---

**Tip:** *Tonight's routine represents a complete evening practice. With these sessions we create an environment for ourselves where our daily observations and emotions can surface so that we may better accept and understand them. Often, insights happen during the rest period after practice, when the mind has been freed from the constraints of the day and the nervous system has been supported in allowing us to recapture a state of ease.*

## Day 5

Longer exhales help us release tension and unwind. Tonight we will apply the 4:8 timing to our evening practice of circular breathing. This morning we will blend the 4:4 timing with breath initiated movement. With practice, this will become second nature.

*Morning Exercise:*

# 4:4 HORIZON BREATH, BREATH INITIATED MOVEMENT

**Total time: 10 minutes**

*Steps*

**1.** Begin your morning practice with the Breath Prep Stretch and Reset Sequence (page 43.) Continue to work with rib cage breathing and resistance breathing. Today, try practicing with your mouth closed. The friction for the breath still resides at the glottis. Be mindful that you don't experience friction at the nostrils. That's called resistance "sniffing."

**2.** Come to standing and prepare for Horizon Breath (page 90).

**3.** Set your timer for 2 minutes and begin. After a few breath cycles, add the 4:4 timing technique we practiced on day 3: Breathe in for 4 counts. Breathe out for 4 counts.

→

**4.** When your timer alerts you that 2 minutes have passed, step your feet closer together and stand still for a moment. Allow your arms to rest alongside your body and relax your shoulders. Take a few normal breaths.

**5.** Set your timer for 3 more minutes and step the feet apart, preparing for Horizon Breath (page 90).

**6.** Combine the 4:4 timing technique with the Breath Initiated Movement technique (page 110).

**7.** When your timer alerts you that 3 minutes have passed, step your feet together and stand quietly for a moment. Observe how you feel.

**8.** Record your practice.

---

**Tip:** *Working for precision in both timing and breath initiated movement requires laser-like focus. The mind becomes completely absorbed in the nuance of the task at hand.*

*Evening Practice:*
# 4:8 CIRCULAR BREATHING, WINDING DOWN

**Total time: 15 to 20 minutes**

Just as a sigh is a gesture of surrender, consciously prolonging exhales supports us in releasing emotional tension that builds up during the day.

## Steps

**1.** Set your timer for 5 minutes and come to a comfortable seated position for the Body Scan and Tension Release (page 52). Tune in to your senses. Tune in to your body. Actively let go of the tension you have collected during the day.

**2.** Adjust your position, stretch your legs, then come back to your sitting posture for circular breathing. Set your timer for 2 minutes. Work through steps 3 through 7 from day 3's evening practice (page 124).

**3.** Set your timer for another 3 minutes, and return to circular breathing.

→

**4.** As you practice, add a 4:8 timing: Count to 4 as you breathe in. Count to 8 as you breathe out. Staying relaxed, continue with the timing until 3 minutes have passed.

**5.** When your timer alerts you that 3 minutes have passed, continue your current cycle, finishing with your next exhale.

**6.** Return to normal breathing and sit quietly for another minute or two. Notice how you feel.

**7.** Choose your favorite resting posture, and lie down for 5 to 10 minutes. After your rest, record your practice.

---

**Tip:** *The 4:8 timing asks for an out breath that is twice as long as the in breath. If the exhale feels too long, try a 4:6 timing. During times of acute anxiety, or in the midst of panic, 4:5 can be a helpful place to start. Slower exhales settle us. Note that when you are counting timings during practice, you have less mental attention available for rambling thoughts.*

## Breath and Emotion: Cultivating Awareness

You are probably familiar with the saying "choke back tears." In order to keep our emotions inside us, we must literally stop our breathing. If expressing emotion is our body's natural way of processing intense experiences, then resisting emotional expression interrupts our ability to fully integrate and move on from the events that cause us duress.

Obviously, it is not appropriate to express our emotions freely in certain settings. If as children, however, we receive messages that there is *never* an appropriate time for emotional release and that expressing our emotions is socially undesirable, dangerous, weak, immature, or shameful, we become experts at subverting them. The result is emotional rigidity and a limited capacity to heal, grow, and trust, which inevitably interferes with our ability to see ourselves and others clearly.

Emotional release is often a precursor to profound personal insight. Free the breath and you free emotion. Certain breathing practices serve to untangle latent emotions that have been expertly kept at bay. It can feel scary to open up to them at first. If you find you have tears in your eyes during practice or you experience other intense emotions, you are not alone. When emotions arise, loosen the reins a little. Trust in your ability to heal from your experiences by allowing your emotions to rise to the surface and literally *move* you.

# Day 6

Though we will continue to vary our morning and evening practices in order to build on our skill set, today's practices represent well-rounded options for an ongoing daily routine. Notice how many techniques you now have in your toolbox that can be combined to form a more complete daily practice.

## *Morning Exercise:*
# BREATH OF FIRE + 4:4 HORIZON BREATHING

**Total time: 20 minutes**

Today we expand our morning practice to include three exercises. Each affects our mind-body in a different way, setting the tone for the day ahead. This morning we follow the breath prep stretch and reset and the enlivening breath of fire with the energizing horizon breath.

## Steps

**1.** Begin your morning practice with the Breath Prep Stretch and Reset Sequence (page 43). Continue to engage with rib cage breathing and resistance breathing. Again, experiment with closing your mouth during resistance breathing. The friction for the breath should still happen at the glottis, not in the nostrils.

**2.** Come to a comfortable seated position for Breath of Fire (page 116). Complete 3 rounds of 12 to 30 breaths per round. (As your practice progresses, gradually work toward 3 rounds of 30 breaths.) Take recovery breaths between rounds. During this rest, check for and release any tension in your body and observe how you feel.

**3.** Come to standing and prepare for Horizon Breath (page 90). Set your timer for 3 minutes and begin. Use rib cage breathing with resistance breathing. Practice breath initiated movement with the 4:4 timing from day 5's practice (page 135).

**4.** When you have finished, come to sitting and rest for a minute or two. Use this time to observe the effects of your breathing practice on mind and mood.

**5.** Record your practice.

---

**Tip:** *Morning practice takes a certain amount of will and determination. Though I hope you are enjoying the ritual, as it becomes less novel you may find that you talk yourself out of doing it. The best way to avoid this daily decision is to put your body in motion. Don't think. Just do.*

# 4:8 ALTERNATE NOSTRIL BREATHING

**Total time: 15 to 20 minutes**

Morning breaths support daytime activities; the evening exercises should lead us toward a good night's sleep. Tonight's practice combines three breathing skills: circular, alternate nostril, and timing.

## Steps

**1.** Come to a comfortable seated position and set your timer for 5 minutes. Practice the Body Scan and Tension Release meditation (page 52).

**2.** When you have finished your scan, stretch your legs and adjust your position in preparation for 3 more minutes of seated breathing practice.

**3.** Set your timer. Close your eyes. Relax your shoulders. Relax your jaw. Completely relax your hands. Begin to take long, smooth breaths.

**4.** Begin with Alternate Nostril Breathing (page 119).

**5.** As you engage with alternate nostril breathing, if it feels natural to do so, incorporate Circular Breathing (page 124).

**6.** Once you feel comfortable and have found your rhythm, begin to assign the following timing to your breath: Breathe in for 4 counts. Breathe out for 8 counts. *Note:* If at any point during your breathing you start to feel agitated, frustrated, or short of breath, simply stop to rest. Wait until you feel ready to start again.

**7.** When your timer alerts you that 3 minutes have passed, continue with the current cycle until you have completed an exhale through your left nostril.

**8.** Release your right hand to your lap and return to normal breathing. Sit quietly for another minute or two. Observe how you feel.

**9.** Lie down on your back and rest for 5 to 10 minutes.

**10.** After your rest, slowly return to sitting and record your practice.

**Tip:** *As mentioned, lengthening the out breath supports the activation of the PNS and helps us resolve our responses to stress. This timing can be incorporated into breathing during any part of the day but is particularly helpful at night when you are trying to wind down. After practice, reflect on the kinds of thoughts you were having (if any) during your practice or during your rest. How were your thoughts paced? Were they images or words?*

# Day 7

Congratulations! Today is the final day of the second week of your journey toward better breathing. Plan a little extra time in your practice this morning for journaling. Tonight, we will do our end-of-week review.

## Morning Exercise:
# 3-MINUTE BASELINE

**Total time: 10 to 15 minutes**

Let's return to our baseline exercise to see how you're doing. This is not a test. It's just an opportunity to gather information.

**1.** Set your timer for 5 minutes. Challenge yourself to take smooth, even resistance breaths as you move through the Breath Prep Stretch and Reset Sequence (page 43). If it does not yet feel natural to practice resistance breathing with the mouth closed, it is fine to continue with the mouth open.

**2.** Come to a comfortable seated position and set your timer for 3 minutes.

**3.** Close your eyes and begin to count your breaths. As before, resist the urge to approach this exercise by actively trying to take fewer breaths. Your only job is to take full, comfortable breaths at a comfortable and easily manageable pace.

## Document your progress

We have now recorded three baselines. Depending on where you started, it's possible you might observe some change. Take a little extra time with your journal this morning to think more broadly about your week so far. Look through the lens of mind and mood. Consider the following questions:

» Has Breathwork helped you become more aware of your thoughts?

» What have you noticed about your emotions this week?

» Is this aspect of the work interesting to you?

» How have you been sleeping?

» What are your fears?

» What are your doubts?

» Is there anything else that has been going on for you that might be worth recording here?

**4.** When your timer alerts you that 3 minutes have passed, make a mental note of how many breaths you've taken. Return to normal breathing. Notice how you feel.

**5.** Open your journal and record the number of breaths you took in 3 minutes. Record any other observations, ideas, or insights worth noting as you wrap up week 2.

# REST AND RESTORE, THE RECLINED BREATH WAVE

**Total time: 15 to 20 minutes**

Time for a break. We will start with journaling so that after our rest and restore practice, we can more easily remain in what I hope will be a delicious, easeful, and relaxed state.

## Steps

**1.** Take 5 minutes to work with your journal. Revisit your weekly log and your assessment of mind and mood from the beginning of week 2. Rate your current experience with the issues you listed. Note any changes.

**2.** Fold your blanket in preparation for the Opening the Chest Reclined Posture (page 42, figure 2.5). Set your timer for 10 minutes. Lie down on your folded blankets. If this position is uncomfortable for you, lie down on your back.

**3.** Allow for natural breathing. Observe the subtle shift of the low back and pelvis as you breathe.

**4.** Transition to belly breathing. Take 3 or 4 Belly Breaths (page 57). Rest for 2 or 3 breaths.

**5.** Once belly breathing is established, explore slightly deeper breaths, encouraging the lower rib cage to join in with your breathing. When you breathe out, imagine your exhale sliding down the back surface of your body toward your toes. Take 3 or 4 belly-to-low-rib-cage breaths. Rest for 2 or 3 breaths.

**6.** Next, take slightly deeper breaths, encouraging the middle chest and side ribs to open to receive each in breath. When you breathe out, imagine your exhale sliding down the back surface of your body toward your toes. Take 3 or 4 belly-to-mid-rib cage breaths. Rest for 2 or 3 breaths.

**7.** This might be a good place to stop. If you feel anxious, agitated or short of breath, skip to step 9.

**8.** Consider 2 to 3 more breath waves. This time, experiment with using your full lung capacity, allowing the upper chest and the space under the collarbones to fill with breath. When you breathe out, imagine your exhale sliding down the back surface of your body toward your toes. One or two belly-to-collarbone breaths might be enough for today.

**9.** When you've finished, rest quietly until your timer alerts you that 10 minutes have passed.

**10.** Exit the posture slowly. Roll off your blanket to one side and draw your knees in toward you. Rest here. When you feel ready, press up to a comfortable seated position and orient yourself to the room. Notice how you feel.

**11.** Before you leave your practice this evening, place a palm over your heart and appreciate the soft rise and fall of your chest as you breathe. Take a moment to cultivate a sense of gratitude for your breath and how it enlivens you every single day.

---

**Tip:** *Keep in mind that progress is not always linear. Perhaps the breathing practices we did this week loosened some carefully held emotions, and you are now feeling moodier or more emotionally fragile than you did before we got started. Don't be concerned; you are resilient.*

# Cultivating Connection

The term *mind-body* is meaningful, but it's not quite complete.
We tend to think of ourselves as a mind, a body, and "a little
something special." Whether you see yourself as infused
with consciousness, spirit, or soul or as a sophisticated,
intelligent machine, anyone with an inquisitive mind would
not hesitate to appreciate the beauty and complexity of the
elements that come together to make a living human being.

As you become more embodied and more aware during practice,
occasionally you will find yourself feeling pleasantly alive, awake,
and rooted in a sense of ease and belonging. In week 3 we will
shift our focus yet again in order to appreciate these spontaneous
and poignant moments that become available to us through
Breathwork. As we shake hands with that little-something-special
part of us, we become curiously present to the fact that we are not
alone but rather intimately connected and richly entangled with
the lives of others and within nature as it unfolds around us.

## Day 1

Today we begin our third and final week of breathing. Plan on spending a little extra time with your journal after this morning's practice, as we will create a new weekly log. Tonight, we will begin to work with briefly suspending our breathing.

*Morning Exercise:*
# COMPLETE MORNING PRACTICE

**Total time: 15 minutes**

From now on we will start most mornings with the breath prep stretch and reset sequence, followed by the breath of fire. In combination with the horizon breath, this morning's practice represents a complete series for ongoing Breathwork.

## Steps

**1.** Begin with the Breath Prep Stretch and Reset Sequence (page 43). Use rib cage breathing and resistance breathing. Breathe with your mouth open or closed during resistance breathing.

**2.** Come to a comfortable seated position for Breath of Fire (page 116). Complete 3 rounds of 12 to 30 breaths. (As your practice progresses, gradually work toward 3 rounds of 30 breaths.) Take recovery breaths between rounds. Check for and release any tension in your body.

**3.** Come to standing and prepare for Horizon Breath (page 90). Set your timer for 3 minutes and begin. Use rib cage breathing with resistance breathing. Practice breath initiated movement with the 4:4 timing from week 2, day 5's practice (page 135). If you choose to breathe with your mouth closed, be mindful that you do not "sniff" the breath in. The sound of resistance breathing comes from your throat, not your nose.

**4.** When you have finished, come to a comfortable seated position and rest for a minute or two. Enjoy the effects of your practice.

**5.** Record your practice.

---

**Tip:** *This week our practices will start to resemble routines I hope you will take forward beyond this 21-day program. As you work with Breathwork in week 3, start to observe which practice combinations are working best for you. Make note in your journal, so you can refer to it as you make decisions moving forward.*

*Evening Practice:*

# SUSPENDING THE BREATH

**Total time: 15 minutes**

In this exercise, we briefly pause our breathing. Remember to stay relaxed as you begin to work with this process. We want to let go of tension, not cause it! Please refer to chapter 2, page 61 for more on the timings and suspensions we will be working with this week.

## Steps

**1.** Come to a comfortable seated position for the Body Scan and Tension Release meditation (page 52). As you get more and more used to this practice, you may not even need to set your timer. Resist the urge to rush, however. Use this time to give your nervous system an opportunity to reintegrate and reorient after the events of your day.

**2.** After your scan, stretch your legs and adjust your position in preparation for seated breathing.

**3.** Set your timer for 3 minutes. Recall the Path of the Breath meditation (page 71) and practice for 8 to 10 breath cycles. If Circular Breathing (page 124) is feeling natural to you, you may use it for this exercise, but it is not essential.

**4.** When you feel ready, continue taking full, smooth breaths. Let your awareness settle on the transition between the end of your inhale, when the lungs are full, and the beginning of your exhale.

**5.** Without closing your glottis, experiment with prolonging the pause between the end of your inhale and the beginning of your exhale. Do not prolong the pause so long that you start to feel short of breath. Think of this more as a "pregnant pause" than an actual holding of your breath.

**6.** Take only one or two suspension breaths at a time, followed by 2 or 3 recovery breaths. Repeat.

**7.** When your timer alerts you that 3 minutes have passed, sit quietly for a moment. Observe how you feel. Consider lying down for 5 to 10 minutes of rest.

**8.** After your rest, return to sitting and record your practice.

---

**Tip:** *If you are feeling apprehensive about this exercise, you are not alone! Many find it causes anxiety to even think about holding the breath. Don't worry. You may adapt this practice to your comfort level. If you are experiencing a more acute state of anxiety or are in the midst of a panic attack, do not try to hold the breath at all. Instead, practice the 4:5 breath timing.*

# Your Weekly Log: Going Deeper

Humans are wired to seek meaning. We are curious about our purpose and want our lives to have relevance. We want to matter. If we wish to use personal practices such as yoga, meditation, or breathing to connect more deeply with a sense of meaning and purpose, we should start by making our intentions explicit.

This week, make a list of the things that you value most in life. What is most meaningful to you? What inspires you? What would you like to see or experience more of? Examples might include fostering connections with others such as partners, parents, children, or friends; pleasurable activities such as spending time in nature; creative pursuits such as cooking or making art; or altruistic impulses such as supporting your family or engaging in service. This list is a draft that you may edit at any time.

Next, list any goals you have for personal growth. These would be areas in your life in which you would like to see lasting change, such as letting go of self-doubt, overcoming a particular fear, or experiencing more intimacy in your relationships. This list may contain things about yourself that are getting in the way of you more regularly enjoying the things you value most.

Next to each *value*, rate on a scale of 1 to 10 how much time and/or attention you devote to the things you value most. Are they currently a small or large part of how you experience your life? Next to each *goal*, rate where you believe yourself to currently be on a scale of 1 to 10, with 10 representing having achieved your goal.

This log is different from the others. The physical act of breathing may not on the surface seem to be directly relevant to these higher ideals, but implementing any well-being practice without looking toward your big-picture goals would represent a missed opportunity. We will revisit this log at the end of the week.

## Day 2

As you explore adding suspensions into your breathing practice, observe how both mind and body become absorbed in the details of the skill you are working to master. Combining suspensions and timings adds a layer of challenge to Breathwork and can serve to amplify the effects of a given breathing exercise.

*Morning Exercise:*

# 4:1:4 HORIZON BREATHING

**Total time: 10 minutes**

This morning's exercise includes a short pause between the in breath and the out breath during horizon breathing.

*Steps*

**1.** Begin your morning practice with the Breath Prep Stretch and Reset Sequence (page 43) for 3 to 5 minutes. Use rib cage breathing and resistance breathing.

**2.** Come to standing, set your timer for 3 minutes, and prepare for Horizon Breath (page 90).

**3.** Take a moment to refine your posture. Check the placement of your feet. They should be wider than hip distance apart, with your toes pointing forward. Bend your knees. Bring your hands together in front of your chest. Softly focus your eyes on something in front of you, or close your eyes.

**4.** Begin horizon breathing. As you practice, add the following 4:1:4 timing to your breath: Count to 4 as you breathe in. Pause for 1 count. Count to 4 as you breathe out.

**5.** When your timer alerts you that 3 minutes have passed, step your feet together and stand quietly for a moment. Observe how you feel. Consider sitting or lying down for a few minutes to rest.

**6.** Record your practice.

---

**Tip:** *The full inhale of the horizon breath encourages an expansive and open rib cage. The brief pause prolongs the sense of vibrancy that is intrinsic to this powerful posture. Suspend the breath when both arms are open and the lungs are at full capacity. Keep your glottis open, and without lifting your shoulders, use this moment to stretch your rib cage as if you are trying to take more breath in. Focus your effort into the side ribs and back ribs as well as into your front chest.*

Evening Exercise:

# 4:4:8 CIRCULAR BREATHING

**Total time: 15 to 20 minutes**

As you play with extending breath suspensions, as in this 4-count pause, keep in mind the duration is simply a suggestion. If 4 counts feel too long, simply make your pause shorter.

## Steps

**1.** Set your timer for 5 minutes and come to a comfortable seated position for the Body Scan and Tension Release meditation (page 52). Tune in to your senses. Tune in to your body. Actively let go of the tension you have collected during the day.

**2.** Adjust your position, stretch your legs, then come back to your sitting posture for Circular Breathing (page 124). Set your timer for 2 minutes and begin.

**3.** When you've finished 2 minutes of circular breathing, set your timer for 3 minutes and practice circular breathing with the 4:4:8 timing: Count to 4 as you breathe in. Pause for 4 counts. Count to 8 as you breathe out.

**4.** When your timer alerts you that 3 minutes have passed, continue with your current cycle until the end of your next exhale.

→

**5.** Return to normal breathing and sit quietly for another minute or two. Notice how you feel.

**6.** Choose your favorite resting posture, and lie down for 5 to 10 minutes. After your rest, slowly return to sitting and record your practice.

---

**Tip:** *The rhythms and repetition of timings are mildly hypnotic and can bring us into a meditative state. If you practice regularly, you may find yourself getting "lost" in the breath. We usually notice these states in retrospect. For example, your timer will ring and rouse you from a pleasant state of simply being.*

## Day 3

As we blend our foundational techniques with timings and suspensions, you may find it helpful to revisit the instructions from previous exercises. This morning we will insert a suspension after each round of the breath of fire. This evening, we will keep it simple and enjoy the balancing effects of alternate nostril breathing.

*Morning Exercise:*

# BREATH OF FIRE WITH RETENTION + CIRCULAR BREATHING

**Total time: 10 minutes**

Fast breathing makes suspending the breath easier temporarily. Notice an enhanced capacity to retain your breath after the breath of fire.

## *Steps*

**1.** Begin your practice with the Breath Prep Stretch and Reset Sequence (page 43). Practice rib cage breathing with resistance breathing for the entire duration of the series.

**2.** Come to a comfortable seated position for 3 rounds of Breath of Fire (page 116). Usually we take recovery breaths after each round. Today, we will suspend the breath. Close your eyes.

→

**3.** Practice 1 round of breath of fire.

**4.** After 12 to 30 breaths, take a long, full breath in. Fill your lungs all the way up to the top. Close your glottis and hold your breath in. Encourage the same sense of suspension you worked with on day 1. All you have to do is pause at the top of the in breath and enjoy the silence, stillness, and fullness of your lungs.

**5.** Whenever you are ready, release your breath, exhaling smoothly. Consider applying a little resistance at the throat to assist the breath out in one long, even release. Draw your belly in at the end of the out breath.

**6.** Now, take 2 or 3 recovery breaths.

**7.** Repeat steps 3 to 6 two more times. When you suspend your breathing, keep the shoulders, jaw, and hands relaxed. Suspend for only as long as is absolutely comfortable and no longer. Release the breath whenever you feel ready.

**8.** After 3 rounds, check again for tension in your body. Sit quietly for a moment. Breathe normally.

**9.** Finish this morning's practice with 5 calming Circular Breaths (page 124). You decide how deep or how subtle to make these breaths. As a way of keeping track, rest the back of your right hand on your right thigh, and use your fingers to count your breaths as you take them.

**10.** After 5 circular breaths, return to normal breathing and once again observe how you feel. Open your eyes.

**11.** Record your practice.

---

**Tip:** *After this morning's practice, pay special attention to your energy level as you move forward with your day. Do you feel lethargic and slow? Do you feel speedy? Our goal is to use our breathing to more regularly feel poised, stable, balanced, and ready for the day ahead. We followed this morning's suspension practice with a few calming circular breaths. How might the end result have been different if you finished with horizon breathing instead?*

*Evening Exercise:*

# ALTERNATE NOSTRIL BREATHING

**Total time: 15 to 20 minutes**

Suspensions and timings can be stimulating, and for some people they can be exceptionally challenging. Tonight, we return to the basics, using alternate nostril breathing to facilitate composure and ease.

## Steps

**1.** Come to a comfortable seated position and set your timer for 5 minutes. Practice the Body Scan and Tension Release meditation (page 52).

**2.** When you have finished your scan, stretch your legs and adjust your position in preparation for 4 minutes of seated breathing practice.

**3.** Set your timer. Close your eyes. Relax your shoulders. Relax your jaw. Completely relax your hands. Take a few long, smooth breaths.

**4.** Begin Circular Breathing (page 124). Take 7 to 10 circular breaths.

**5.** Add alternate nostril breathing, beginning with an exhale through the left nostril as described on page 132.

**6.** When your timer alerts you that 4 minutes have passed, continue through the cycle until you find yourself exhaling through your left nostril.

**7.** Release your right hand to your lap and return to normal breathing. Sit quietly for another minute or two. Observe how you feel.

**8.** Set your timer for 5 to 10 minutes and come into the Reclined Resting Pose (page 38).

**9.** When your timer alerts you, slowly return to sitting. Record your practice.

---

**Tip:** *You may find that more often than not you require no more than a simple, no-frills practice such as this one. It is often during the rest after practice, whether we remain seated or lie down, that we feel most connected to that little-something-special part of us. Consider using these moments to recall the things that are most meaningful to you—the values you wrote down in your weekly log—as a way of spending a little time with them each day.*

## Day 4

Today is a special day! Not only are we passing the halfway point of week 3, we will establish our voice with the exultant "ha!" breath. I am also including an optional bonus afternoon practice, which is a wonderful option for that time of day when you find your energy and focus starting to wane.

## *Morning Exercise:*
# "HA!" BREATH

**Total time: 10 minutes**

There is something tremendously freeing about this vocalization. However, if there are others sleeping peacefully in your home, you'll need to save it for later.

## Steps

**1.** Begin your practice with the Breath Prep Stretch and Reset Sequence (page 43). Practice rib cage breathing with resistance breathing. Use this time to play with the closed-mouth version of resistance breathing.

**2.** Come to standing, set your timer for 2 minutes, and prepare for 4:1:4 Horizon Breathing (page 157). It varies for everyone, but if you prefer to count breaths rather than use your timer, 2 minutes should be around 12 to 15 breaths.

**3.** When you've finished 2 minutes of breathing, step your feet closer together and rest for a few breaths.

**4.** When you're ready, step your feet apart as you would in preparation for horizon breathing. Take your arms out to your sides, with your elbows slightly bent and your palms facing up. Tip your chest up toward the ceiling slightly and lift your gaze.

**5.** Open your mouth, draw your belly in, and take a big, full, fast rib cage breath in. When you exhale, blast the air out and shout, "ha!"

**6.** Repeat, taking anywhere from 8 to 24 "ha!" breaths.

**7.** After your breaths, step your feet closer together for several recovery breaths. You may also sit or lie down. Notice how you feel.

**8.** Record your practice.

---

**Tip:** *Each practice represents an opportunity to intentionally engage with your purpose. The "ha!" breath disrupts your internal status quo. You might even find yourself giggling afterward. Ask yourself the question, "Am I holding anything back?" If you feel lightheaded after this breath, simply bend your knees, rest your forearms on your thighs, and put your head down. The feeling should quickly pass.*

*Optional Afternoon Exercise:*
# THE BOX BREATH

**Total time: 3 minutes**

Navy SEALs are taught this simple breath to hone clarity and focus. Not only can it help you reorient when you're distracted, it can also give you an edge before activities that require sharp attention. Note that this breath incorporates a suspension after the out breath.

## Steps

**1.** Find a fairly quiet and comfortable place to sit where you won't be interrupted for a few minutes. This could be at your desk, in your car, or under a tree in the park.

**2.** Set your timer for 2 minutes. Sit tall and relax your shoulders. Choose a comfortable breathing pace for the 4:4:4:4 (box breath) timing: Count to 4 as you breathe in. Pause for 4 counts. Count to 4 as you breathe out. Pause for 4 counts.

**3.** Continue with this timing until your timer alerts you that 2 minutes have passed. Return to normal breathing.

**4.** Slowly open your eyes and take in the room around you. Observe how you feel.

*Evening Practice:*

# SUSPENDING THE BREATH + OPENING THE CHEST RECLINED POSTURE

**Total time: 15 to 20 minutes**

If you practiced the box breath this afternoon, you may have noticed that inserting a pause after your out breath felt very different from the suspensions we've explored up until now. Let's continue exploring what it's like to suspend our breathing when the lungs are empty.

## Steps

**1.** We will start with seated practice and end with the Opening the Chest Reclined Posture (see page 42, figure 2.5). Set up your folded blankets, so the support will be waiting for you when you're ready to lie down later.

**2.** Set your timer for 5 minutes. Begin with the Body Scan and Tension Release meditation (page 52).

**3.** When your timer alerts you that 5 minutes have passed, adjust your position, stretch your legs, then come back to a comfortable seated position.

→

## Steps (cont.)

**4.** Set your timer for 3 minutes. Recall the Path of the Breath meditation (page 71) and practice for 8 to 10 breath cycles. If Circular Breathing (page 124) is feeling natural to you, you may use it for this exercise, but it is not essential.

**5.** When you feel ready, continue taking full, smooth breaths. Let your awareness settle on the transition between the end of your exhale, when the lungs are empty, and the beginning of your inhale.

**6.** Without closing your glottis, experiment with prolonging the pause between the end of your exhale and the beginning of your inhale. Do not prolong the pause so long that you start to feel short of breath. Like before, think of this more as a "pregnant pause" than an actual holding of your breath.

**7.** Take only 1 or 2 suspension breaths at a time, followed by 2 or 3 recovery breaths. Repeat.

**8.** When your timer alerts you that 3 minutes have passed, sit quietly for a moment. Observe how you feel.

**9.** Set your timer for another 5 to 10 minutes. Lie down on your support. Ensure that your head is supported and your arms are away from your body. Rest.

**10.** After your rest, roll off your support to one side, and return to sitting. Record your practice.

---

**Tip:** *When something shocks us emotionally, we might place a hand over our heart, exhale, and pause for a moment with the lungs empty, as if to mark the relevance of the moment. Afterward, we tend to breathe more fully, as if remembering the fragility and tenderness we embody so casually most of the time. You may have noticed it is more challenging to hold your breath when your lungs are empty. Work on staying relaxed during this kind of exploration.*

# Day 5

As I mentioned in chapter 1, Breathwork is not prescriptive. However, even though we've been integrating new skills this week, you have probably been noticing there is a pattern to our practices. This morning we will work with circular breathing; tomorrow we will work with horizon breathing. Our evenings are generally simpler and include a rest.

*Morning Exercise:*

# BREATH OF FIRE
# WITH RETENTION +
# CIRCULAR BREATHING

**Total time: 10 minutes**

In the stillness of your pauses, when the lungs are full, enjoy the sense of satiation that occurs after your in breath.

**1.** Begin your practice with the Breath Prep Stretch and Reset Sequence (page 43). Practice rib cage breathing with resistance breathing for the duration of the series.

**2.** Come to a comfortable seated position in preparation for 3 rounds of Breath of Fire with Retention (page 161).

**3.** After each round, fill your lungs to capacity and hold your breath in. Exhale smoothly. Follow with 2 or 3 recovery breaths.

**4.** After your third round, sit quietly for a moment. Breathe normally. Release any tension in your body.

**5.** Move on to Circular Breathing (page 124). Take 5 to 10 circular breaths.

**6.** Sit quietly and observe how you feel.

**7.** Record your practice.

---

**Tip:** *Suspending the breath when the lungs are full could be seen as an act of savoring abundance. You are effectively prolonging the feeling of having satisfied your need for breath. On the other hand, suspending when the lungs are empty could be seen as an act of trust. We are invited into the stillness of emptiness and must trust that another breath will come.*

# Evening Exercise:
# COMPLETE EVENING PRACTICE

**Total time: 15 to 20 minutes**

Return to this basic evening routine regularly. This routine reinforces integration, establishes awareness, and, with the inclusion of step 8, invites us to revisit our highest intention. Consider this practice a complete evening sequence for ongoing Breathwork.

## Steps

**1.** Come to a comfortable seated position, and set your timer for 5 minutes. Practice the Body Scan and Tension Release meditation (page 52).

**2.** When you have finished your scan, stretch your legs and adjust your position in preparation for 4 minutes of seated breathing practice.

**3.** Set your timer. Establish a relaxed state in preparation for Circular Breathing (page 124).

**4.** Take 7 to 10 circular breaths. Then, add alternate nostril breathing to circular breathing. Begin with an out breath through the left nostril as described on page 132.

**5.** When your timer alerts you that 4 minutes have passed, continue through the cycle until you find yourself exhaling through your left nostril.

**6.** Release your right hand to your lap and return to normal breathing. Sit quietly for another minute or two.

**7.** If you are sitting comfortably, feel free to stay in this position for a few more minutes. Alternately, lie down on your back and rest.

**8.** During your rest, consider the following inquiries: Scan through your body and notice any physical sensations. Observe your mind and notice any thoughts, images, or words. Check in with your emotions. Extend your awareness to include everything outside of your body. Become aware of the room you are in, people nearby, objects, other buildings, nature, water, sky . . . nothing is off limits. To finish, bring your awareness back to your breath, and focus your mind on what is most meaningful to you.

---

**Tip:** *Going, going, going without stopping, the way so many of us live our lives, does not allow for introspection. Whether during the poignant moments between breaths or during the longer pauses after practice, Breathwork can awaken you to yourself, others, nature, and your sense of purpose.*

# Breath and Flow: Cultivating Connection

Recall a memory from your childhood where you had the experience of being completely absorbed in something. Perhaps you lost yourself in the building of a block tower, or you forgot the world for a little while when gazing up at the clouds. Maybe you remember a moment of elation on your bicycle with the wind whistling in your ears, or you found yourself completely absorbed in a drawing. When you were a child, this compelling state of mental focus was a natural part of everyday play.

Psychologist and researcher Mihaly Csikszentmihalyi describes this pleasurable experience of becoming fully immersed in the activity at hand as a state of *flow*. As adults, our busy lives limit the opportunities for stumbling into flow. Our culture invites us to rush from one thing to another. We squeeze things into our day and have grown tolerant of being pressed for time. Though the practices of Breathwork are short, the final two or three minutes—the time when you pause to observe the effects of the practice—are perhaps the most important. It is in that window, should you allow for it, that you might find yourself spontaneously easing into a certain kind of quiet alertness, heightened awareness, or even uninhibited joy. Soothed and awake, you are finally able to sit comfortably within yourself and enjoy moments where you can clearly see that we are all connected and whole.

## Day 6

It can be helpful to have a qualified teacher make choices for you about your practice. Teachers take into account aspects of personality, lifestyle, and skill level and can guess which practices might bring you more growth. However, for practice to remain consistent, you need to enjoy it. In the absence of a teacher, craft your routine around the practices you feel drawn to, and trust in your innate ability to know what is best for you. You can always change your mind.

### Morning Exercise:
# BREATH OF FIRE + 4:1:4 HORIZON BREATHING

**Total time: 10 minutes**

Repetition is integral to developing mastery. After week 3 you could choose to work with today's morning sequence for a while or with yesterday morning's practice.

### Steps

**1.** Begin with the Breath Prep Stretch and Reset Sequence (page 43). Use rib cage breathing and resistance breathing. Breathe with your mouth open or closed during resistance breathing.

→

**2.** Come to a comfortable seated position for Breath of Fire (page 116). Complete 3 rounds of 12 to 30 breaths. (As your practice progresses, gradually work toward 3 rounds of 30 breaths.) Take recovery breaths between rounds. Continue to check for and release any tension in your body.

**3.** Rest for a few breath cycles. Observe how you feel.

**4.** Come to standing and prepare for Horizon Breath (page 90). Set your timer for 3 minutes and begin. Use rib cage breathing with resistance breathing. Practice breath initiated movement with the 4:1:4 timing from day 2 this week (page 157).

**5.** When you have finished, come to a comfortable seated position and rest for a minute or two. Enjoy the effects of your practice.

---

**Tip:** *During yesterday morning's practice, we incorporated breath suspension after the breath of fire and followed with circular breathing. This morning, we inserted the pause during the horizon breath. Have you developed a preference?*

*Evening Practice:*
# 4:8:4 CIRCULAR BREATHING

**Total time: 15 to 20 minutes**

Tonight, our circular breathing practice includes a timing that incorporates breath retention after our out breath. It's possible that you may not yet feel ready for this step. Give yourself permission to work with one of the previous day's versions of circular breathing. You can always come back to this timing later.

## Steps

**1.** Set your timer for 5 minutes and come to a comfortable seated position for the Body Scan and Tension Release meditation (page 52). Tune in to your senses. Tune in to your body. Actively let go of any tension you have collected during your day.

**2.** Adjust your position, stretch your legs, then come back to your sitting posture for Circular Breathing (page 124). Set your timer for 2 minutes and begin.

**3.** When you've finished 2 minutes of circular breathing, set your timer for 3 minutes and practice circular breathing with the 4:8:4 timing: Count to 4 as you breathe in. Count to 8 as you breathe out. Pause for 4 counts.

**4.** If you are in the middle of a breath cycle when your timer sounds, finish your current cycle, ending with your next exhale. →

**5.** Return to normal breathing and sit quietly for another minute or two. Notice how you feel.

**6.** Choose your favorite resting posture, and rest for 5 to 10 minutes.

**7.** Record your practice.

---

**Tip:** *We have been discussing using breathing to access that little-something-special part of ourselves. Perhaps breath suspensions are intriguing because when we are able to comfortably sustain them, they most resemble that state of quiet alertness we associate with flow.*

## Day 7

You have done it! Today marks 21 days of continuous Breathwork. Take a moment to absorb it and celebrate. Plan a little extra time around your morning and evening practices for journaling. We will revisit not only this week's weekly log but also your logs from week 1 and week 2.

*Morning Exercise:*
# 3-MINUTE BASELINE

**Total time: 10 to 15 minutes**

Today we return to our baseline to see how far we've come. After 20 days of consistent practice, it is now reasonable to look for progress.

## Steps

**1.** Set your timer for 5 minutes. Observe your breathing as you move through the Breath Prep Stretch and Reset Sequence (page 43).

**2.** Come to a comfortable seated position, ready your timer, and prepare for the 3-Minute Baseline (page 12).

**3.** Take long, full, comfortable breaths, counting the breaths as they pass, until your timer sounds. Do not strain in an effort to slow your breathing. Rather, as best as you can, *enjoy* your breath, as if you don't want to miss anything about it.

**4.** Pull out your journal and record the number of breaths you took in 3 minutes.

→

## Journal: Documenting Your Progress

If you have been committed to this work, you most likely have seen progress in your baseline. However, slowing the breath is not the goal in and of itself. Rather, a slower breathing rate is an indication of improved efficiency and an enhanced capacity to remain continuously engaged with your breathing. We have now recorded four baselines. Have you noticed a change? Take a little extra time with your journal this morning to think more broadly about this week. Look through the lens of overall well-being. Consider the following questions:

» Has Breathwork helped you feel more connected to yourself and/ or to others?

» Do you feel more or less in touch with a personal sense of meaning or purpose?

» Is this aspect of the work interesting to you?

» How have you been sleeping?

» What are your fears?

» What are your doubts?

» Is there anything else that has been going on for you that might be worth writing down here?

*Evening Exercise:*

# 4:7:8 BREATH + REST AND RESTORE WITH LEGS UP THE WALL

**Total time: 20 minutes**

For our final practice together, we will work with the rest-inducing 4:7:8 timing. Start with journaling so that after your seated breathing you can settle into a deep rest and restore relaxation.

## Steps

**1.** Take 5 minutes to work with your journal. Revisit your weekly logs from all 3 weeks. Rate your *current* experience with the issues you listed each week, and note any changes. This exercise is intended to help you evaluate the areas in which you are experiencing perceived progress, whether subtle or dramatic, after 3 weeks of Breathwork.

**2.** When you've finished journaling, set up for seated breathing practice near a wall or chair.

**3.** Come to a comfortable seated position for circular breathing. Set your timer for 3 minutes. Relax your shoulders. Relax your face. Completely relax your jaw. Don't forget to relax your hands, too. Sit a little taller and take 5 to 7 Belly Breaths (page 57).

**4.** Once belly breathing is established, ease into Circular Breathing (page 124). As you are ready, apply the 4:7:8 timing: Count to 4 as you breathe in. Pause for 7 counts. Count to 8 as you breathe out. Continue with this timing until your timer alerts you that 3 minutes have passed.

**5.** Now set your timer for 10 minutes. Lie down on your back with your legs up the wall (see page 106, figure 3.6.). It is easiest to enter this posture from a seated position with one hip touching the wall.

**6.** If this posture puts a strain on your low back or your knees, or if you are using muscular effort in your legs to stay in this position, it will not feel restful. Instead, use a chair. See figure 3.7 (page 106).

**7.** Allow your arms to rest away from your body. Move your shoulders down and away from your ears. Close your eyes.

**8.** Bring your awareness to your breath. Notice which parts of your body move naturally when you breathe in this position. Observe the subtle rocking of the pelvis, the sense of elongation and contraction of the spine, and the expanding and narrowing of the rib cage with each breath cycle.

**9.** Each time you notice your mind wandering, gently and without judgment call it back to your breathing. If you start to drift off to sleep, allow it. This position is a wonderful one in which to enjoy a prolonged rest.

**10.** When your timer alerts you that 10 minutes have passed, slowly draw your knees into your chest, roll to one side, and return to a comfortable seated position. Take another minute or two to orient yourself to the room. Observe how you feel.

**11.** Before you leave your practice this evening, place a palm over your heart and appreciate the soft rise and fall of your chest as you breathe. Take a moment to cultivate a sense of gratitude for your breath and how it enlivens you every single day. Open your journal and record the last practice of your 21 days of Breathwork.

---

**Tip:** *The 4:7:8 timing is particularly conducive to rest. It can be practiced while sitting or even lying down in bed in preparation for sleep. Use this breath when the mind is racing and you are having a hard time winding down. If you suffer from low back pain, regularly incorporate the deeply restful legs up the wall pose into your practice. Over the last 3 weeks you have gathered three resting poses for your toolbox: reclined resting pose, opening the chest reclined posture, and legs up the wall pose.*

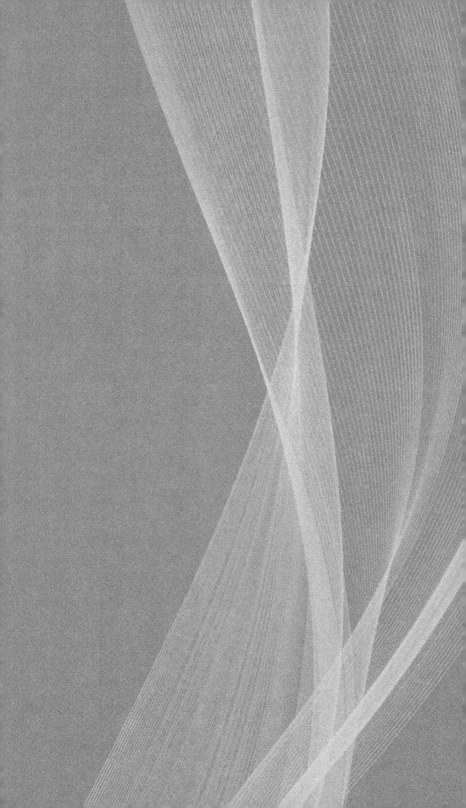

# Conclusion
# A Tool for Everyone

In the last 21 days, we have discovered that the way we breathe can affect us profoundly. Using our breathing, we can address bodily sensations including pain, enhance or deplete certain chemical balances, and increase or decrease our aptitude for producing energy. Our breathing can help us build and enhance neural connections, unearth and heal old hurts, and help us override autonomic nervous system reactions. We have learned that our breathing can support us in experiencing pleasure and connecting with others. Our breathing practice can even serve as a gateway to a sense of pleasant absorption we might otherwise experience during deep meditation or activities that bring us into a state of flow. The question that needs to be answered now is whether Breathwork has been useful for you and, if so, how you would like to continue.

Though it's easy to appreciate the ways in which we instinctively use our breathing, such as when we laugh, sob, sigh, form words, exercise, or sing, we cannot escape that we are born into a culture that teaches us to look outside of ourselves for answers and that trains us to transcend the capacity of our physical bodies, often at the expense of our own health and well-being.

I'll give you an example. It is healthier to walk to work every day than it is to ride on a train or drive a car. However, technology affords us the ability to live farther from our workplaces than we could if we did not have access to transportation. Now, we hold the stress of timing our travel—in order not to be late—in our bodies. Our bodies also hold the stress of navigating to our destination, remaining vigilant and alert during our journey. Meanwhile our bodies are sedentary, and our breathing is shallow.

This is not how we were designed. We were made to move and breathe our way through the very physical activities that, up until recently, were required of human beings for survival. Our bodies were designed to participate fully, and this would have traditionally included regular and dramatic changes to our breathing rate, style, and volume throughout our day.

If our work and play do not provide us with the amount of physical stress our bodies need to stay healthy, we have learned we must artificially replicate it with exercise. Given what we know about breathing and its importance to physiological homeostasis, psychological health, and overall well-being, it's entirely possible that expressive and varied breathing patterns are equally important to replicate.

Each breathing exercise presents an opportunity to shift something in you. Staying present to the effects of each practice and taking the time to notice how you feel is the key to discovering how to engage with your breath moving forward. Breathwork is here to serve you. Consider it a gift. Let it support you in all that you are.

## Guidelines for Ongoing Practice

Below are my suggested guidelines for ongoing practice.

» If a given practice feels like too much in any way, simply do less. Sometimes you can feel lightheaded or develop a headache after practice. This would be an indication that you either did too much too fast or you chose an exercise that wasn't right for your very individual internal ecosystem at the time.

## Special Journal: Wrapping Up

You did it. Take a moment to let it soak in. For our final journal exercise, reflect on your experience with Breathwork overall. It's all too easy to forget where you were when you began, but your journal has a fair amount of history in it now. Read through your journal entries and make note of the key areas in which Breathwork has been impactful for you so far. Next, look over your weekly logs. With these entries you have created a personal profile that describes where you feel you are currently around things that matter to you, such as your physical and emotional health, as well as for your higher aspirations for a more meaningful life. You have also documented where you would like to see change. The exercise alone has served to make what may have been implicit goals explicit. Finally, take a few minutes to think about the work you've been doing. Here are some questions to consider:

» Did you come to Breathwork for a particular reason?

» Were you true to the program?

» Did Breathwork serve to address a particular concern?

» Did Breathwork affect you in ways you didn't expect?

» Do you think continuing with this work would benefit you? If so, how?

» How would you like to continue with Breathwork?

» Record any other thoughts, ideas, concerns, or observations that occur to you.

» If a given practice left you feeling wonderful, grounded, focused, vibrant, and clear-headed, stick with that practice until it loses its potency.

» Establish a regular routine. Practice once or twice a day. Practice at least three days per week. Five or six days is ideal.

» Choose one to three exercises that you feel drawn to continuing. Remember that once you settle on a routine that works for you, you do not need to vary it as often as we have been doing these last weeks. Over time and with consistent practice, your agency with the techniques will build, and your comfort level will grow. It's fine to repeat what works for you.

» When you become bored or feel ready for a change, come back to this program and start again. Inevitably you will learn in layers. Incorporate the exercises or variations that you didn't feel ready to work with before or excluded for other reasons. Regularly go back to the basics.

» Experiment. Just because you didn't like something the first time, that doesn't mean you shouldn't continue to experiment with it, learn more about it, inquire into its purpose, vary it to suit you, or otherwise come into a process of exploration.

» Emotional release is normal. It should not be seen as an indication that you should stop or change a particular practice but rather as a sign that the practice is working to help you move through difficult emotions. In most cases the content behind the emotional release will become clear and over time will lose its charge.

» Regular, repetitive, and intense emotional release or strong, unpleasant emotions or moods that linger after practice, become unmanageable, or become amplified with practice should be taken seriously. If this happens, discontinue your practice until you can speak to your care provider, and seek the help of a professional before continuing.

## Building Your Personalized Practice

Deciding to practice every day is a wonderful goal. However, follow-through can be a challenge. Maintaining an ongoing personal practice is hard. We need to break it into smaller chunks. Here are some suggestions for building your personalized practice.

**1.** Pick a time frame. Set yourself up to bring your breathing practice forward for a designated, doable period of time: Ours was 21 days; yours could be four weeks, three months, or a season. Commit now. Challenge yourself to put your practices in your calendar and treat them as important and not to be missed.

**2.** Choose a practice. The simplest thing to do would be to flip back to week 1 and start Breathwork again. You will experience the work differently the second time through. You will have access to developed nuance and skill, and you will probably amplify your results. Alternately you may use the suggested examples of complete breathing practices from week 2 and week 3 (pages 132, 140, 142, 152, 172, 174, and 177). Or you can customize your own practice.

**3.** Regularly include the Breath Prep Stretch and Reset Sequence (page 43) or another gentle movement sequence. This sequence releases tension and loosens the body in preparation for breathing. I have included this sequence in the morning routine, but it may be done before evening practice as well.

**4.** Regularly include the Body Scan and Tension Release meditation (page 52). There are many ancillary benefits to including this meditation. Besides cultivating awareness, improving mental focus, and releasing tension in preparation for breathing, the body scan engages the different regions of the brain, promoting integration, and brings awareness to unconscious physical tension patterns in the body that may need to be resolved for efficient breathing.

**5.** Sandwich one or two Breathwork exercises per practice between the breath prep stretch and reset sequence or the body scan meditation as modeled in weeks 1 to 3 and a short seated or reclined rest. Recall suggestions for complete breathing practices from week 2 and week 3.

**6.** Generally, choose stimulating exercises during morning practices. These include fast breathing and/or rib cage breathing and certain timings as presented in weeks 2 and 3. These can be followed with calming or more balancing exercises.

**7.** Generally, choose calming and relaxing practices during evening sessions. These incorporate belly breathing or circular breathing and certain timings as presented in weeks 2 and 3, so as not to disturb the potential for restful sleep.

**8.** Finish each practice with a brief self-awareness assessment and/ or rest. An honest daily self-assessment of the physical, emotional, and overall effects of your breathing practice is key to developing an understanding of how to steer your practice in the right direction. If you regularly feel physically uncomfortable or otherwise disturbed after practice, this may be an indication that you are doing too much. Enhanced clarity, ease, relief, and joy are all signs that you are on the right track.

# What's Next?

If you're wondering what's next after Breathwork, entertain the possibility that you will not exhaust the practices in this book. I have been working with the breathing exercises presented here for more than 20 years. My favorite exercises remain, without question, the most basic ones from week 1. However, as you develop mastery, you may find yourself looking for something a little different.

You are walking away from these 21 days with a solid understanding of the eight types of foundational breathing exercises. Anything that you pick up "out there" will be a variation of one of these eight breathing types. There is nothing wrong with experimenting with variations. Innovation in this field continues, so keep exploring. I look forward to breathing with you into the future.

# Additional Resources

## Books

*Anatomy of Breathing.* Blandine Calais-Germain, Eastland Press; 1st ed. (December 4, 2006).

*The Breathing Book: Good Health and Vitality through Essential Breath Work.* Donna Farhi, Holt Paperbacks; 1st ed. (November 15, 1996).

*A Life Worth Breathing: A Yoga Master's Handbook of Strength, Grace, and Healing.* Max Strom, Skyhorse; 1st ed. (April 7, 2010).

*Self-Awakening Yoga: The Expansion of Consciousness through the Body's Own Wisdom.* Don Stapleton, PhD, Healing Arts Press; PAP/COM edition. (July 22, 2004).

*Yoga: The Spirit and Practice of Moving into Stillness.* Erich Schiffmann and Trish O'Reilly, Pocket Books; 1st ed. (December 1, 1996).

## Websites

The American Institute of Stress, https://www.stress.org/

American Thoracic Society, https://www.thoracic.org/

Chest Foundation, https://foundation.chestnet.org/

Luma Yoga, Inc., https://lumayoga.com

# Courses and Online Content

Ancient Yoga, Vedic Philosophy, Tantra courses available at Shuklacharya.com

Chakra Theory and Meditation, Online Course with Paul Grilley, Pranamaya.com/courses/chakra-theory-and-meditation

Inner Axis Method and Breathe to Heal courses available at MaxStrom.com/inner-axis

Strategic Breathing App for Anxiety and Stress, iTunes.Apple.com/us/app/strategic-breathing/id1273620853?mt=8

# References

Block, Richard A., David P. Arnott, Barbara Quigley, and Wesley C. Lynch. "Unilateral Nostril Breathing Influences Lateralized Cognitive Performance." *Brain and Cognition* 9, no. 2 (1989): 181–90.

Craig, A. D. "Forebrain Emotional Asymmetry: A Neuroanatomical Basis?" *Trends in Cognitive Sciences* 9, no. 12 (2005): 566–71.

Craig, Bud. "How Do You Feel? Lecture by Bud Craig," December 14, 2009, Video, 1:03:25. https://vimeo.com/8170544.

Csikszentmihalyi, Mihaly. "Flow and the psychology of discovery and invention." HarperPerennial, New York 39 (1997).

Dallam, George M., Steve R. McClaran, Daniel G. Cox, and Carol P. Foust. "Effect of Nasal Versus Oral Breathing on Vo2max and Physiological Economy in Recreational Runners Following an Extended Period Spent Using Nasally Restricted Breathing." *International Journal of Kinesiology and Sports Science* 6, no. 2 (2018): 22–29.

Hakked, Chirag Sunil, Ragavendrasamy Balakrishnan, and Manjunath Nandi Krishnamurthy. "Yogic Breathing Practices Improve Lung Functions of Competitive Young Swimmers." *Journal of Ayurveda and Integrative Medicine* 8, no. 2 (2017): 99–104.

Karam, Marilyn, Bani P. Kaur, and Alan P. Baptist. "A Modified Breathing Exercise Program for Asthma Is Easy to Perform and Effective." *Journal of Asthma* 54, no. 2 (2017): 217–22.

Keeler, Jason R., Edward A. Roth, Brittany L. Neuser, John M. Spitsbergen, Daniel James Maxwell Waters, and John-Mary Vianney. "The Neurochemistry and Social Flow of Singing: Bonding and Oxytocin." *Frontiers in Human Neuroscience* 9 (2015): 518.

Lundberg, J. O., G. Settergren, S. Gelinder, J. M. Lundberg, K. Alving, and E. Weitzberg. "Inhalation of Nasally Derived Nitric Oxide Modulates Pulmonary Function in Humans." *Acta Physiologica Scandinavica* 158, no. 4 (1996): 343–47.

Pal, Gopal Krushna, Ankit Agarwal, Shanmugavel Karthik, Pravati Pal, and Nivedita Nanda. "Slow Yogic Breathing Through Right and Left Nostril Influences Sympathovagal Balance, Heart Rate Variability, and Cardiovascular Risks in Young Adults." *North American Journal of Medical Sciences* 6, no. 3 (2014): 145.

Pratt, Laura A., Debra J. Brody, and Qiuping Gu. "Antidepressant Use among Persons Aged 12 and Over: United States, 2011-2014. NCHS Data Brief. Number 283." National Center for Health Statistics, 2017.

Reddy, M. S. "Depression: The Disorder and the Burden." *Indian Journal of Psychological Medicine* 32, no. 1 (2010): 1.

Simon, Lee S. "Relieving Pain in America: A Blueprint for Transforming Prevention, Care, Education, and Research." *Journal of Pain & Palliative Care Pharmacotherapy* 26, no. 2 (2012): 197-98.

World Health Organization. *Depression and Other Common Mental Disorders: Global Health Estimates.* No. WHO/MSD/MER/2017.2. World Health Organization, 2017.

# Index

*Timings (Continued)*

# Acknowledgments

I give enduring love and gratitude to my dear husband, Nick, who has been absolutely unwavering in his encouragement, support, and belief in me over the years. I am grateful for my daughters, Poppy and Amma. You are my teachers. Really. I am grateful, and I love you.

Love and thanks to all generations of my family for your ever-present love, patience, and goodwill. Especially I thank Jujie, for feeding us and driving kids around, but mostly for your friendship.

Deepest gratitude for my teachers, including my dear mentor and friend Max Strom, who continues to inspire me, and Shukl'acharya Shree, with whom I had the privilege of deeply engaging with daily pranayama practice as well as connecting, through his ardor, to the profound and soulful roots of devotional yoga. You are both with me in my teaching and every time I practice. Love and thanks to Denise Kaufman and Paul Grilley for giving me permission to throw out the rulebook and replace it with logic, innovation, and play.

Thanks to my dear friends and colleagues Julie Gallant, Kyra Haglund, Teya Hardy, Vivica Shwartz, and Giselle Tsering. You are patient with me, and you give me courage.

I give thanks to my business partners and soul sisters Lynda Meeder and Kate Tripp for believing in me. Kate, the gift of your professional eye has been invaluable. I am grateful. And I thank all the brilliant and capable souls who have kept our business purring along while I stepped away to dive into Breathwork, including Kaysi Contreras, Leanna Immel, Shannon Jenkins, Sasha Neese, and Amy Rawlings. Nina Hoffer, you saved me in the eleventh hour.

Sincere appreciation to Callisto Media for the opportunity to rise to the occasion.

Most humbly, I thank my students, who have trusted me with their valuable time and allowed me to experiment and grow over the years. You think you are the student, but in reality, it is I who am learning from you every day.

# About the Author

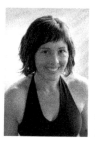

**Valerie Moselle** is an advanced yoga teacher and founder of Luma Yoga, an award-winning yoga studio and wellness center in Santa Cruz, California. She is the creator and lead instructor of the Luma Yoga Teacher Training program. A twenty-year veteran of teaching yoga and Breathwork, Valerie has taught alongside industry leaders including Shiva Rae, Seane Corn, and Eric Schiffman. She is known for classes that inspire a playful exploration of breath, movement, strength, and surrender.

A student of yoga for nearly three decades, Valerie has studied and taught in the San Francisco Bay Area, Southern California, India, and the United Kingdom. She works in close collaboration with international *Breathe to Heal* teacher Max Strom to coach teachers around the world.

Valerie currently lives with her husband and two daughters in Santa Cruz, where she serves as the director of Luma Yoga, Inc.

CPSIA information can be obtained
at www.ICGtesting.com
Printed in the USA
BVHW090122230519
548808BV00001B/1/P